Pebbles in the Water

A New Collection

by
B. LEWIS BARNETT, JR., M.D.

Professor Emeritus and Founding Chair
Department of Family Medicine
University of Virginia School of Medicine

For more information on the Society of Teachers of Family Medicine Foundation visit:
www.stfm.org/foundation/index.html

ISBN: 1-58597-222-3

Library of Congress Control Number: 2003112559

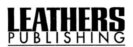

A division of Squire Publishers, Inc.
4500 College Blvd.
Leawood, KS 66211
1/888/888-7696
www.leatherspublishing.com

To Annalyne,
my beloved wife and companion,
who lived through these stories with me.

And to the patients who
have allowed me to share their stories.

ENDORSEMENTS FOR DR. BARNETT'S WORK

I have known Dr. Lewis Barnett for nearly thirty years. To say I have been a student of his for many years would be an understatement, because in addition to being my teacher, he has also been my family's doctor, my patient, my colleague and my very good friend. He has been a constant guide in the lives of countless students, residents and patients. He has influenced my life and career since the first time we met in Charleston, South Carolina. I was a first year resident in Family Medicine; it was a hot humid July day in 1974. My wife and I had just moved to Charleston and not yet unpacked all our belongings. The night before my first day of training, we had been "rear ended" at a traffic light by an intoxicated sailor from the Charleston Navy Base. The news of the accident had made its way to Dr. Barnett. We had never met; my time with the residency had just begun — this was my first official day! Lewis made a point of finding me that first morning, and after making sure that no one was seriously injured in the accident and in need of his immediate help, he let me know that he was available if I needed anything. All I needed to do was ask. He then handed me a piece of paper with his home telephone number. "Just call, anytime." I still have his home phone number, and I still call at all hours of the day and night. It is good to know that he is there ready to be helpful.

Pebbles in the Water is the second collection of Dr. Barnett's thoughts, stories and poems. It comes at a time in his life when most "professors" are retired and no longer teaching. Yet these true stories are as contemporary as "morning report" on an inpatient family medicine service. They reflect the knowledge, feelings, thoughts and experiences that most family doctors have, but fail to notice during a hectic day. These stories go beyond the interpretation of the latest MRI scan or laboratory report. They describe the true art of healing. Dr Barnett teaches that the art of medicine begins first and foremost with knowledge, but must pull extensively on the doctor's ability to connect with the patient and to apply the knowledge in such a way that healing can occur. Dr. Barnett eloquently shares his experiences in a manner that gives flesh to the textbook knowledge — allowing the reader to see beyond the disease to understand the patient and, most importantly, to see into the heart of one extraordinary physician.

Each small chapter in this book is full of the love, grace and joy this remarkable teacher and family doctor has demonstrated to his many students and patients for over fifty years. I have a favorite photograph showing me as a young resident examining a patient. Standing in the corner of the examining room, observing and silently cheering me on, is Lewis Barnett. I will always be grateful to Lewis for "being in my corner," whether physically present or not.

I know that Lewis Barnett is symbolically present in the corner of countless exam rooms. The family doctors he has touched during his extraordinary career are scattered across the country and number in the hundreds! Each doctor knows that all he or she needs to do is pick up a phone and Lewis is ready to help.

Each of these stories — pebbles — helps to uncover and describe the soul of Family Medicine, forming an indelible image of the true Family Physician. Read them slowly, and learn from them the importance of the doctor patient relationship. It is this privileged connection between the patient and the doctor that allows healing to begin. As Dr Barnett writes and has taught for many years:

- Do more than exist; live
- Do more than look; observe
- Do more than listen; grasp
- Do more than touch; feel
- Do more than hear; understand
- Do more than think; ponder
- Do more than talk; say something.

— *John J. Collins, M.D.*
Grand Rapids, Michigan

Over the years, I have been blessed to meet and know a number of people who are, by all objective and subjective standards, "great men" or "great women." Lewis Barnett is clearly in this category, and this is apparent early to most who meet him. What may not be so definable is the reason for this greatness. Now, through his stories and insights, others can experience what those closest to him are moved by. There is no guile, no pomp, no veneer; just a clear view of a man's heart and soul dedicated to serving not only humanity, but most of all, the single human person in need.

His gift for healing and for exhorting comes from the center of a secure soul that has nothing to hide or to be afraid of. He allows human weaknesses and hurts to come forth not as glaring "warts on a nose," but as old associates that need some understanding.

All of these stories have the same basis — a man reflecting on his life as a healer — but each one is as fresh and instructive as a new friendship. To Lewis, that's what they are. Lewis Barnett opens up human hearts because, just like the front door of his home, *his* heart is always open.

— *Andy MacFarlan, M.D.*
Practicing Family Physician
Earlysville, Virginia
(Former resident of Dr. Barnett)

As long as I've known him, Dr. Barnett has told stories. I remember many Sunday afternoons after "Sunday lunch," and late nights when I just needed to talk, that Dr. B. and I would discuss patients, medicine and life. He'd often tell a story to make a point: stories of how he dealt with his own insecurities as a doctor, stories of difficult patients, stories of how patients had touched him. As I read his newest book while visiting Dr. and Mrs. B. up on the mountain, my mind wandered back to his darkly paneled office in Charlottesville, decorated with Western art, keepsakes from patients, students and residents, and the red phone. The red phone was designed not to call heads of state, but to receive urgent calls from students and residents who needed to talk. Dr. Barnett shared easily, insightfully and genuinely.

I realize now, much like a son unconsciously develops the habits of his father, how I have consciously or unconsciously caught some of the habits of my mentor. Greeting a patient with "There you are" is something I have made a practice of doing. Only recently, in re-reading Dr. Barnett's first book, did I realize that I learned this salutation from him. There is much to be "caught" from Dr. Barnett. His newest book, *Pebbles in the Water*, is a compilation of such stories — true experiences in which something significant, sometimes even eternal, happens. Through these vignettes, Dr. Barnett demonstrates that what has been given is far greater than he can give. His capacity to give does not arise from some innate strength or sense of duty. It comes from a sense of gratitude that has become a "spring of water welling up" (John 4:15), refreshing him and those around him.

Read thoughtfully. I hope you will catch a glimpse of what I observed firsthand as one of Dr. B's "ripples in the pond."

— *David J. Schriemer, M.D.*
Practicing Family Physician
Vicksburg, Michigan

For six decades, even before he was Dr. Barnett, I have known Lewis Barnett as college classmate and close friend. Then he became my family's physician and my parishioner. His medical career has mirrored or excelled the best I have ever known of. He is an almost uncanny and gifted diagnostician, a compassionate family practitioner, a faithful and caring teacher. Thousands have felt his healing touch and presence and, thankfully, multiplied thousands will be blessed through those whom he has taught.

— *Rev. Victor Adair Greene*
Retired Minister and
Missionary to the Philippines
Greenville, South Carolina

CONTENTS

Preface xiii

1. Pebbles, Quietly Making a Difference 1
2. Toad 5
3. An Unseen Star 7
4. A Sip of Water 11
5. The Last Field Trial 13
6. Invisible Sutures 17
7. Fabulous Fawn 19
8. In the Clouds 23
9. Anne Valeece 25
10. Acquaintance with the Night 29
11. The 'Iffy' Places 31
12. Hiram and the Leaking Boat 33
13. A Comb 35
14. Snapshot Mentality 37
15. Lesson from Hurricane Hugo 39
    Down by the Creek 41
16. The Dirty Needle 43
17. The Way We Remember 45
18. Four Outfits 47
19. At the Women's Social 51
20. In Another's Moccasins 53
21. Bigotry and Bias 55
22. If Physicians Are Artists 57
23. Defining Legacy 59
24. Brightly Colored Afghan 61
25. The Rusty Scupper 65
26. Miss Becky's Second Fashion Show 67
27. Dear Mary Waddell 69
28. Special Delivery 73
29. What Christ Means in My Daily Work 77
30. I'm Coming 79
31. Wonder Why That Is 81
32. Who's In There? 85
33. Put Them Through, Dora 87

34.	E Pluribus Unum	91
35.	Touching a Toe	93
36.	I Ran Away	97
37.	You Can't Help Me	99
38.	If You Are So Inclined	101
39.	Breast Lump	103
40.	I Can See	105
41.	Dean of Women	109
42.	Blue Concrete	111
43.	Splendor Intensified	113
44.	In Search of Flander's Ointment	115
45.	Human Splint	117
46.	Peaks and Valleys	119
47.	Prognosis in Perspective	123
48.	In Whatever Way I Can	127
49.	She's Never Been	131
50.	The Night the Brakes Went Out	133
51.	Artist in Overalls	135
	Marriage	137
	What Love Is Not	139
52.	May Day	141
53.	The Dancing Girl	147
54.	The Only One	149
55.	Therapeusis of a Rocker	151
56.	Fireworks	153
57.	The Anvil Stands	155
58.	While Eating Supper	157
59.	Water Marked	159
	Watching the Sunrise	161
60.	Benjamin	163
61.	Writing in the Margins	165
62.	One January Night	167
63.	Candle in the Wind	169
	Life Cycle: Autumn, Now Winter	171
64.	Like Joseph's Coat	173
65.	Nostalgic Aroma	175
66.	Feelings of the Heart	177
67.	Roller Coasters	179
	Melody of Life	181

68. The Eyebrows Said Yes 183
    Trustee of Dreams 185
69. Wren at My Window 187
70. You're a Keeper, My Friend 189
    It's Okay to Cry 191
71. On the Doorstep 193
72. Ode to the Stethoscope 195
73. Bill's Symphony 197
74. Yeah, I'd Jump Again 199

PREFACE TO THE SECOND COLLECTION

Some thirteen years ago, my first collection of true stories was published under the title *Between the Lines*. The fact that it is still available and is being read even now makes me realize that true stories often resonate with those who have had similar feelings and experiences. Often a true story awakens that precious experience long forgotten. Now I add another collection of stories, no less true than the first, hoping that they will enhance memories in your own lives of very significant experiences.

In trying to come up with a name for this second collection, I came across an anonymous poem.

> *Do a deed of simple kindness,*
> *though its end you may not see.*
> *It may reach, like widening ripples,*
> *even to eternity.*
>
> —*Anon.*

Then I ran across a second anonymous saying. It conveyed almost the same sentiments.

> *Drop a pebble in the water,*
> *just a splash and it's gone;*
> *But there's half a hundred ripples*
> *circling on and on and on.*
> *Circling outward from the center,*
> *circling outward to the sea,*
> *till there's no earthly way of knowing*
> *where the end is going to be.*

xiii

I chose pebbles instead of stones because this collection of stories deals with the little things, the subtle moments, the fine print of one man's reminiscences, not the headlines.

With these thoughts in mind, I decided to call these new stories *Pebbles in the Water*, hoping that each story will encourage you to toss your pebble into the water too.

—B. Lewis Barnett, Jr., M.D.
4734 Talleybrook Drive, N.W.
Kennesaw, Georgia 30152

One

Pebbles ... Quietly Making a Difference

Since I began medical school in 1945, and you can do your math, I have been walking the walk of a family physician. First I practiced in my small hometown for a period of two decades, then answered the call into academe where I spent the next thirty-two years. At no time was I willing to give up practicing, seeing my own patients as well as seeing patients with generations of family practice residents. From the beginning, my life has been dedicated to seeing one patient at a time, doing the best I knew how at the time, with the knowledge that I had at that particular time. These fifty-seven years have brought a kaleidoscopic chain of events that have literally changed our world. We find ourselves reaching into a new millennium, which presents a moving target. Still we will be expected to be there for those who are sick and compromised as their hope and help for coping with illnesses and stresses brought on by a frenzied society with new and uncommon demands. Regular illnesses are now wound tightly with an intense wrapping of invisible, choking twine. This makes diagnoses more difficult to ascertain. The real problem is sometimes hidden beneath layer after layer of overlying situational stresses. Such intricate mysteries walk into our doors crying for help — not knowing which lyrics to put to their soulful song. We are often baffled and discouraged.

Dr. Denis Burkit once said, "Not everything that counts can be counted." We might say it another way, that we tend

1

to measure only that which is measurable. So much of what creates the essence of our existence is in the realm of intangibles. The air we breathe we can not see. Some things we take for granted. Each person, physician or patient, lives in a world all their own. Often each feels very much alone, even in a crowd. True stories become the hallmark of every physician's encounter with life as he or she experiences it. We become the interpreters of, and the participant in, the biographies that we touch. I know that those in our profession who are led to be totally scientific may view anecdotal evidence with suspicion. However, the truth is, as human beings, we live in a world of stories, and since every life is unique, each story of necessity will not be exactly replicable in another life. As our patients reveal their stories, their secrets, they often purge themselves of the serious emotional malignancies that taint and ruin their quality of life. For physicians to listen is perhaps the most basic therapeutic tool we have to offer. The question for us today is what has happened to rob us of that precious gift? Not one of us should relish rushing through patient visits so fast that all the patient gets from us is our own preconceived notions about what they might have come for. How can we create an atmosphere where patients can feel safe enough to open their hearts a little wider, so that we are invited into the intimate and secret parts of their biographies that would make our diagnostic efforts more accurate from the outset? This would require a trusting relationship. In other words it would require the restoration of a covenant between two trusting souls — each believing in the other.

A dedicated doctor's life, indeed every day of it, is filled with often once in a lifetime opportunities — occasions to touch outcomes with unique hands and heart — maybe never again — but today — this time — now — is the time to do something very special for this person. I try to, as I believe we all can, walk into each room with that feeling that something special may be about to take place. Listen for the story, wait for that feeling of coupling. It takes no longer to listen intently than it does to ignore; no longer to give 100% of yourself than it does to give 50%. The days can be a series of wonderfully interesting short stories — our lives as physicians are interwoven into the fabric of another person's attempt to cope with life — and we are there.

Having said all of this, I now invite you to take a glimpse into my world of stories, one biography at a time. Each one of these vignettes has a point to make. I hope that these true stories will rekindle your thoughts about some of your own experiences. The title, *Pebbles in the Water*, pictures each of us on the banks of a quiet lake tossing tiny pebbles, creating ever enlarging concentric circles on its surface. Each small effort, each interaction with each person sets into motion an ever enlarging effect on the quality of life for those we touch. One, then another, and another — multiplied by as many as we are allowed the privilege of touching — could have a major impact on our world — one person at a time. It could start here — now. I have given each one of these stories a title — each one stands alone and represents one pebble thrown into the water.

Two

Toad

My maternal grandmother's maiden name was Etolia Antho Jane Carnell. Then she married a man named Reid Skinner. So just add Skinner to the aforementioned maiden name. Is it any wonder that her family and friends simplified the matter and called her "Toad" for short. She was quite an unusual lady. Perhaps she was one of the most powerful shaping influences of my young life. It is my belief that the seeds that brought forth the burning passion for medicine in my childish fantasies were sown at her bedside.

I never saw her out of bed in my life. She had been bedridden since before I was born. No one ever told me exactly why she was there or just why she could not get out of bed, or why she could not walk like everybody else. As a child, I could not figure it all out. Why couldn't the doctor cure her? In my naivete, I am told that I made such remarks as, "When I grow up, I'm going to be a doctor and I am going to cure Granny." Of course, she and I never had any formal discourse on the matter.

As I grew up and went away to college, I took pre-med courses at Furman University. Later I was admitted to the Medical College of South Carolina in Charleston. The more I learned, the more I began to surmise what had happened to my "Toad." I believe that she was put to bed because she probably had tuberculosis, together with what was described as "Change of life issues of bleeding." Anyway, over time the chronic illness and inactivity had caused her joints to freeze. Her body had become stiff and gnarled.

When we went to visit her every Sunday, I was always impressed with her pleasant countenance — a perpetual smile — a gentle and kind voice. Her bed was always so clean, the sheets were so white. I later learned that in all of the thirty-two years, there had never been a bed sore. All of this is a tribute to my Aunt Lottie who dedicated her life to caring for her mother. Lottie deserves a story all about such dedication.

After internship at the Protestant Episcopal Hospital of Philadelphia, I returned to my hometown Woodruff, South Carolina and set up practice in the rear of Anderson's Drug Store.

Now the little fellow who had spent his whole life looking up at the tall bed that "Toad" was confined to was now her doctor, much too late to cure her, of course. There would be no more doctor bills for her, ever again. That was my great pleasure.

One night (or more correctly morning since it was 5 a.m.) while making a house call to see the wife of one of the ministers in town, that last call came. "You had better come to Granny's. She is asking for you." I quickly dismissed myself and went straightaway to her house on Allen Street. As I sat down beside her bed, she opened her eyes and asked, "Am I about gone?" I did not answer as I was placing the stethoscope on her chest. Many family members stood around the room in silence. I listened, and as I was listening, I heard the last heartbeat. When that "next" heartbeat never came, I laid the stethoscope aside and placed my ear to her chest. It was over. Thirty-two bedfast years. Such a classy lady, powerful in such a quiet way, influencing by her unique example, defining patience in fresh ways every time I saw her. "Toad" left a grandson who, because of her, has spent over fifty years in medicine. Even though I never saw her walk physically, she stands tall in my memory. Her legacy is indelible.

Three

An Unseen Star

Some days in practice often stretched into the night. Such was this one. The office had been filled with standing room only patients until late, and then there were house calls to make. Spring rains had begun to fall toward night and increased in severity as time went on. Along near the stroke of midnight I was making my last call of the day/night. As I recall, it was to see the Gossett family who lived down near the bottom land around the South Tyger River. The roads down to the river were not paved. The rains continued, the sky was dark, devoid of stars or a moon.

I made it down to the house and found a dim light on the porch. Several members of the family were sick. After tending to all, I fastened my black bag and bid them goodnight. The muddy road proved to be a challenge as the return trip was uphill, not downhill. The car began to slide in and out of ruts previously dug into the red clay of upper South Carolina. About a mile up, I felt the car begin to slide, ever nearer to the edge of a very deep ravine (I call it a gully). The harder I tried to steer it away, the more it seemed that there was a magnet pulling the car ever closer to falling off the road into the ditch. I turned off the switch, sat there in despair. The sky was pitch black, the rains came down in torrents. I could expect no one to be traveling that road tonight. I saw no way out except to start walking.

The only light I had was from a pen light that I kept in my shirt pocket to look down patients' throats. I knew that it would not help to walk down, because the family was all sick there, so I stumbled up the hill, just hoping that the batteries in the little pen light would hold out. After struggling, slipping, and at times falling to my knees, I finally recognized a familiar crossroad, and it was PAVED. The darkness prevailed. After another mile or so, I recognized a mailbox. It belonged to the Galloways. They were friends and patients, but the house was dark, the yard full of barking dogs. I was hesitant to bother them, but I was desperate. Trying not to let the dogs feel my anxiety, I reached the porch and knocked on the door. Nothing happened. I knocked again. Finally, the porch light came on, with a deep voice asking, "Who is it?"

After assuring him that I was who I said I was, Dick Galloway opened the door to find me standing there, with not a dry thread on me, in need of a friend. He invited me in. Most of the other family members still slept, as I recall. I explained what my predicament was. He said, "Never mind. I'll just get the tractor out and we will get you out."

After hearing the sputtering engine from the barn, I went out to join him. We both rode the tractor, still in the black, rainy night, to the site where my car sat helpless with a mean tilt toward the precipice. Dick was a very talented man and was definitely the hero tonight. We, or better said, he successfully negotiated the task at hand, and out we came.

I am recalling this night after a span of about forty years. An indelible memory was born that night. The Gossetts never knew. Dick is now in Heaven. One of the stars in his crown is the one we couldn't see that night. Even the Magi saw a star; I found one without even seeing it.

ART OF MEDICINE

9 a.m.: Patient anxious, pulse 127
10 a.m.: Patient calm, pulse 76
Rx. Used: Compassionate understanding

Thank you

From grateful patient

Four

A Sip of Water

I was working in our rural satellite practice at Nellysford, Virginia when the rescue squad brought in a dear woman who was struggling for breath. Her real name was Margaret Loving. She was in extremis from severe heart disease. The next day was her birthday, but her knowing look told me that she did not believe she would make it till then. We gave many medications to little avail. After all of that, I sat and held her hand, feeling gently for a pulse. I leaned over and asked, "What else can I do for you now? If I can do one thing now, what would you wish?" Softly came the words (almost in a whisper), "a sip of water." I quickly turned around and ran a cup of water from the tap and placed the cup to her parched lips. She took two or three sips with difficulty between breaths, then burped. "Excuse me," she said.

Somehow, wrapped up in this simple, tough moment was a softness that embodies the point that I came here to make. It is sometimes the tiny, subtle, shared moments between physician and patient that make the strongest of statements — that life in our profession is worth living — under any system, however hard others may try to strip it of the personal touch. Just being there when another person needs us will always give fulfillment and peace about what we are doing. This defines our purpose.

Five

The Last Field Trials

My partner, Dr. Armond Stokes (Bill) Pearson always introduced himself as A.S. Pearson, one "S" please!' His best friend was my dentist, Dr. C. Dixon Falls. I make no pretense of using false names here. These two men were inseparable, and their common bond was that they were both avid foxhunters. In fact, Dr. Bill was president of the National Foxhunters Association this particular year.

On a beautiful Sunday morning, Dr. Bill was taking a shower, getting ready for church, when he suddenly collapsed. His wife frantically called me to come quickly. Fortunately, I had not yet left home for church. When I arrived, I found him unconscious. His body was slick from soap suds. This made it all but impossible for me to get a hold on his body, but she and I somehow managed to move him to his bed. His breathing was labored. Other colleagues arrived one by one. The vigil, which was to last three days, commenced. On Wednesday, his respiratory efforts ceased. He was gone. The cause of death was a massive cerebral hemorrhage. I was with him until the end. He was 62. It was hard to let go.

His best friend, Dr. Falls, and I were pallbearers. Our grief made the load feel heavier than if he had not been our friend. I worried because I could see that his friend was faltering.

The following week was hard. There were many other sick people who needed attention. Some of them were his own patients, some were mine. I did my best, while having daydreams of times that my old partner had made encouraging remarks in times of stress through the years. He was always there to give anesthesia for my deliveries. I remembered the time when I was so worried about a delivery. The patient was of small dimensions. I expressed my frustration aloud. In his calm and quiet demeanor he said, "I've never seen one stay in there yet. Bantam hens USUALLY lay bantam eggs!" Releasing my tension, the baby did indeed come out. I was the serious younger, less experienced partner. He was the light-hearted, more mellow one. I missed him.

As the week went on, every night after finishing up making house calls, I would think about Dr. Bill's grieving friend. This one night I had a strong sense that I should turn up the street where Dr. Falls lived on the corner. Although it was almost ten o'clock, I would drop by to check to see how he was doing (if the lights were still on.) Just as I rounded the corner the lights went off, so I passed on by and headed for home.

The next day was Thursday and I was in the middle of a busy time in the office. I was seeing Linda Metcalf when Dora, my trusted receptionist, interrupted. Ms. Falls was on the phone, "It's urgent." Dora had a way of knowing by the tone of voice just when to interrupt me. Her usual stoic nature had turned to panic. "Come, Lewis, Doc just passed out across the bed." He had just been home for lunch when this happened. Having had a sort of premonition the night before, I feared the worst. I left Linda sitting there and bounded down the hall and out the side door.

Not stopping for traffic lights, I got to their house in no time, only to find Ms. Falls standing at the door holding the screen open for me. Her distraught countenance was obvious as she exclaimed, "I'm afraid you're too late. He's not breathing." On examination, he was pulseless and breathless. (Fortunately, just a few weeks before I had attended a seminar where Dr. James Jude from Hopkins had discussed his paper on *Closed Chest Cardiac Massage.*) Dr. Falls turned out to be my first "save." After mouth-to-mouth resuscitation and chest compressions for an eternity, it seemed, he exhibited opisthotonic motions (decerebrate rigidity) and gasped for breath. So shocked was I that I involuntarily jumped back. Some of my colleagues had answered Mrs. Falls' call to the hospital for help. Lynn Long, the technician, had brought oxygen and the EKG machine. I feared that his brain had been without oxygen too long. Some said that was true. In spite of the naysayers, I kept up my efforts. It just would have been too much to lose these two prominent figures within nine days.

Transported to a large hospital about twenty-five miles distant, he remained unresponsive for four days. He had been restrained by placing a fishnet apparatus over the railings on the bed. He picked at the netting for a time, until finally he opened his eyes. He began to talk. He told this incredible story about having seen "Bill." They had been at the National Field Trials that took place in Camden the week before. He and Dr. Bill had reservations before he died. Somehow, the two great friends had connected in these stress-torn days. He said, "We had a real good time. He was happy."

Dr. Falls was my dentist for three more years. He returned to his practice and was his "normal self." He did a major reconstruction of my neglected teeth, and I remember the laboriously tedious hours he worked in my mouth. I kept thinking, not wanting him to overtax himself. My mind raced, "This man was dead. How strange this is."

He never remembered, nor did his wife tell him, what I had done. All he remembered was being at the Field Trials with his friend Bill, who had died just days before the trials took place, and they had such a great time together.

Two great friends. I was fortunate to know them both.

15

Six

Invisible Sutures

I am sitting on the mountain, looking out at nothing but clouds again. It is unusual to have so many days in the clouds during the month of October. The fabled October sky is present only in memories of other years. Such times breed introspection. Just now the major thoughts going through my head have to do with one of my favorite subjects — the healing process — just where does it begin — and what makes it happen? Over the many years of sharing time and space in my examining room with so many different kinds of people with widely divergent problems, I have had cause to wonder about what enhances the healing process. To be sure, a correct diagnosis and assessment of just what is going on is the key element.

Today, it seems to be clearer than ever that those who come in burdened down with secrets and concerns never before exposed, privately held, never told — are often sick because of them. Certainly, whatever pathology they have is magnified by their emotions and attitudes about such pathology. Burdens they have borne alone till now — heavy indeed. Given a trusted doctor and a trusting patient and the safety that is inherent in such a relationship, much unfolding of mysteries begins. As burdens and apprehensions are shared, little by little, they become attenuated by this division — having opened up and "handed" them over to someone else.

Paul Tournier, the noted Swiss physician, once explained this time as a non-surgical, psychological opening, not cutting flesh, but opening nevertheless. Such is a time for exposing "the cancer" and removing it, whatever "it" is — then laying "it" aside and leaving it behind. The doctor can "close" the wound much as a surgeon sutures an incision. Such sutures are invisible.

Regardless of the particular pathology, or rather one's perception of the consequences, there needs to be a sharing (opening up) and dividing the weight of such burdens, then closing them with invisible sutures. All of this requires a physician who has the capacity to understand the other person's fears about what will happen if they do share. During such vulnerable times, they must feel reassurance that their secrets will be handled personally and delicately. Together, they will find and feel strength.

Seven

Fabulous Fawn

Today I saw Juliette, one of my ninety-year-old patients. Somehow there was a different look about her on this particular day. Her hair bespoke of a very recent session with the hairdresser — a slightly different color and sheen than usual as I had remembered. Her countenance was glowing. She did not complain as much nor as loudly as usual.

"What color is it today?" I asked as I reached to touch her hair very gently (of course). She smiled and said, "Fabulous Fawn — with a little blond thrown in; my hairdresser is marvelous. She is such a wonderful person." I replied understandingly, "I can tell."

She had *forgotten* her cane today. I simply sat and observed this *new* creature. Our conversation drifted over into some of the things that were important to her now. Prime among them was Mr. Brannigan, her beau. Mr. B had just had eye surgery for cataracts, and now she exclaimed, "He can really see me, and I wouldn't want to scare him away." I chimed in to say, "So that's what Fabulous Fawn with a little blond thrown in is all about." We both had a good laugh. Consensus abounded.

I realized that we had just been privileged to touch humanity once again. What a blessing it was for her and for me. There were no new prescriptions written this day.

She arose from her chair without assistance and up the hall she went. Fabulous!

*The soul would have no rainbows
if the eyes had no tears.*

Eight

In the Clouds

This morning I woke up on the mountain, 3200 feet above sea level, shrouded with clouds so much that I could not see the "million dollar" view that is visible on a clear day. Our little cabin in the sky has been the incubator for many, many memories.

When you are here, you tend to put life into its proper perspective. When the sun shines and the clouds are missing, you can see several ranges of tall mountains and a little town in the valley (Old Fort). Your vision stretches to a distant beacon light seventy miles away. You have your own private observatory — billions upon billions of stars. You are connected to the universe in a strangely private way — this is your world.

But today, the clouds are all around you, the dampness grips and reaches close to the bone. You sip on the second cup of coffee, looking out the picture window, but there is no view of the mountains. Suddenly you turn your chair to face your partner of forty-three years, just out of the shower, and realize that she is beautiful — inside and out — and you return to thoughts of what really matters in all of this. The view and warmth of the partner at your side far outweighs what you can see outside when the sun shines. This is what endures, even when the clouds creep in and surround you.

Nine

Anne Valeece

This book would not be complete without introducing you to one of the most benevolent people I ever knew. Her name is Anne Valeece, a jolly and kind woman who was the head nurse on Pediatrics at the Episcopal Hospital in Philadelphia where I interned.

I was a Southern boy who had never been that far north before. I had never been to a city as big as Philadelphia before. I didn't know that towns had more than one train station, so when the conductor yelled "Philadelphia," I got off at the Thirtieth Street Station. My one steamer trunk with ALL of my belongings was put off at the Broad Street Station. We both should have gotten off at the North Philadelphia Station. What a mess! I felt alone in a strange world.

I made one call to the Hospital number. Connie Miller, the switchboard operator, came on and said something like "Piscubul hospitul" real fast. I said, "Huh?" She repeated the exact same thing. I told her my predicament. She said, "Where are ya, dearie?" I tried to tell her that I just got off at the first train station. She knew exactly where I was, but I didn't. Anyway, she directed me to look outside and see if I could find a train up in the sky — the "Ell." Of course, I asked, "Whaaaat?" She then told me to catch the "Ell" and get off at Kensington, then look up and you will see the tower of "Piscubul." Finally I did all that Connie told me and there it was, the Tower of dear old Episcopal Hospital. I had no trunk, no clothes except for the ones on my back.

That is where Anne Valeece came into the picture. At that moment she looked like an angel; later she proved that she was one indeed. Throughout the year she acted much like Mother Teresa to several of us interns, who were so often weary, sleep deprived, bedraggled, and penniless. Interns were not paid a stipend in those days, just a bed and lamb stew on Fridays. I hated lamb stew. Anne was just about the best cook in all of Philadelphia, and she was very, very kind. She lived at 3030 North Front Street in one of the typical row houses, easy walking distance from the hospital.

I can still smell the aroma coming from her kitchen. My favorite recipe was "Muscatel Chicken." This book would not be complete if I didn't give you her secret recipe. She would batter and fry the chicken, mostly thighs, in a well-used skillet until it was brown. Then came the secret. She would pour all of the excess grease out until not a drop was left. Then she would pour about two ounces, maybe three, of cheap Muscatel wine into the skillet. This created quite a show, the steam and all. Then she covered it up with a lid that was just the right size. After a bit, the alcohol would evaporate and the sugar from the grapes would, as she would say, "caramelize" the chicken. Well, it tasted like crispy candy, and did it ever fill a hollow spot.

She liked me for some reason. Maybe it started when I was on "her" pediatric ward. There was a little eleven-year-old girl admitted with a tummy ache, possible appendicitis. The admitting doctor had alerted the surgeon. After I examined her, the abdomen just didn't feel rigid enough for me to go along with the diagnosis of appendicitis. I was puzzled. I sat down and stared at the chart until Anne came by and put her hand on my shoulder. Her question, "What's the matter, Lewie?" I confided to her that I was about to clash with the other resident, because I didn't agree that the little patient had appendicitis. I really thought if we waited the night out, she might begin her menses. Anne said, "If you believe that, write it down and sign it." So I wrote, " Possible Menarche." Of course, this was not a usual diagnosis on the Pediatric Ward. The next day, Dr. Pratt came in for rounds. My little patient obliged me — she began the first of many monthly events. From that time Anne not only liked me, but she thought I was a pretty good doctor. I needed that.

Ten

Acquaintance with the Night

After over fifty years of practicing medicine, I have seen and felt and heard many things. I was sitting with a group of young doctors the other day, and all of a sudden it came to me that their biggest problem was dealing with the night calls. I sat and pondered about the night. I remembered patients who became more fearful in the dark. Symptoms seemed to become exaggerated and ominous at night. Sleep deprivation for doctors and for patients creates a subpar functional existence for both.

I thought back to some of the nights, going through the country on house calls and waiting for the stork to arrive … Such solitary journeys brought thoughts of many other problems that keep people awake at night. It was strange, but as I sat there, my memory carried me to more mellow feelings about the night. Somehow the night can become your friend, even though sleep deprivation seems to be an enemy. It seems to me that sometimes one can think clearer, think more globally and can feel ownership of one's space when it is quiet, when most of the world sleeps. The world belongs to you at night. There are fewer distractions. The stars come out against the background of darkness. The mind is set free and there is an elevated quality to silence. You are alone, yet maybe you are not really alone. Peace is here, less cluttered by others.

So it occurred to me that it was time to talk about the night and one's attitude toward it. So many folks spend much time awake in the dark. We need to learn how to make darkness a friend and not an enemy.

Eleven

The 'Iffy' Places

Beverly was, and still is, an unforgettable, very classy lady. She was an extremely talented pianist. Her home had to be constructed with a big enough room to house two Steinway Grand pianos intertwined back to back. She was plagued with many serious circulatory problems. She had been a heavy smoker for many, many years. Her arteries had turned into calcified conduits. Studies showed that she had universal circulatory problems. She had required several surgeries, both carotids and both femoral arteries had obstructions. After one of her more serious surgeries, I went to see her in the recovery room. She recognized me and smiled while she gripped my hand in appreciation. I continued to visit her as she recovered. I never will forget that she repeatedly thanked me for being close when she was in the "iffy places." I had never thought of it, but she labeled those lonely, frightening times as "iffy places." We all have been there, but just didn't know what to call them. They are times when we are not in control, not "in charge." She was in the hands of very competent surgeons, but they were not as familiar to her as the family doctor was. It is important for the family doctor to be there in the "iffy places."

Another special person named Paul comes to mind. I met him on the first week of medical school when he presented himself in my office and asked if I would be his advisor. He was from New York. We became friends and had a wholesome teacher-student relationship. After four years he graduated and went into the Navy. After his tour of duty was over, he went into practice in a town about 65 miles south of Charlottesville.

One Saturday afternoon he was mowing his lawn when the machine took an erratic turn and his right foot was caught underneath it. Three toes were severed. He was brought to the University hospital. He had always been "the Emergency physician," now he was the "Emergency." I went into the emergency room where he was lying and out of habit I took hold of his hand. We were silent, took long looks at each other, but connected. After a little while he said, "I never wanted to be touched before, but I needed to be touched now. Thanks."

Two dear people, in the "iffy places." Not a good place to be alone or with strangers. A very good place for family doctors to be.

Twelve

Hiram and the Leaking Boat

In the early summer of 1970, as I was considering taking a position on the faculty at my alma mater in Charleston, Annalyne and I were being entertained by Dr. Hiram Curry and his wife Marilyn. Hiram was the chairman of the newly created Department of Family Practice. He was Professor of Neurology, so he felt that he needed a few doctors from the hinterlands to act as role models. At least, that is what he said. I felt very much out of place as I walked the halls of academe. In his effort to make the environs of Charleston more enticing, he invited me down to his dock. There he showed me a rather antiquated wooden sailboat. One thing led to another and he said, "I haven't been sailing in quite awhile, let's take a little sail." This country boy had not been around water any bigger than the shoals of the muddy Enoree River, much less what seemed to be the choppy waters of the huge Cooper River. But to be a good sport, I said okay.

After putting the boat in the water, we both got in. I immediately noticed that there was a bucket in the boat. That didn't make me feel so well. As we went away from the shore, I noticed that the boat was taking on water. I knew enough to know that water "inside" a boat can't be very good. I mentioned this to Hiram. In a very seaworthy-sounding voice, he said, "Oh, when the boards get wet they will swell, and the hole will close!" Just in case though, he handed me the bucket and told me if I would feel better, I could bail the water out until the hole closed. This I did, but I was losing the battle and Hiram knew that I was. He grabbed the bucket and started bailing faster, faster, faster — and in his frenzy he threw the bucket out into the Cooper River. With this, he said we'd better try to make it back to shore. "Come about," he yelled as the sails swung around, nearly causing me to go overboard. They barely missed my head. All of this made me yearn for the muddy waters of lesser magnitude.

Our wives welcomed us with open arms, fearing that we were not very good sailors. Annalyne knew I certainly was not. That turned out to be my first sailing experience, and my last, even though we would live "on the water" for the next seven years, NOT "in the water."

I certainly have appreciated every day of life more since that day.

Thirteen

A Comb

Page Booker, a very distinguished, silver-haired Professor of Pediatrics, was a very special kindred spirit. During our many meaningful conversations, each often knew what the other would say next. Have you ever had a friend like that? Well, he was also my patient. If you know how hard it is for one physician to trust another, you can understand how much I cherished his confidence.

I was out having dinner with my colleagues from Roanoke at the Aberdeen Barn when my pager went off. Dr. Booker's dear wife had found him comatose on the kitchen floor. (They had met when he was a medical student and she was a nurse.) I quickly excused myself and went straight to the emergency room. He was undergoing a CT Scan when I arrived. Minutes, then hours, passed. Our vigil continued. His diagnosis was elusive. He had not had a stroke. Nevertheless, he remained comatose. Over many weeks, he never returned to his sharp, distinguished, normal former self.

One day as I was making rounds, I went into Dr. Booker's room. He had been restless and was half-uncovered and exposed, in his own world, disheveled, unkempt and in need of a shave. I could think of no remedy or of anything that I had ever been taught that would be therapeutic in the least.

Almost instinctively, I reached into my shirt pocket and pulled out a small black comb that I habitually carry. I gently combed his hair. When I left the room, he was covered. His countenance was tranquil. It was almost as though he had felt the little comb lovingly finding its way through his tousled hair. When I mentioned this experience to his wife, we wondered if he could have understood the humble intent.

Some years later I was visiting with his widow. She was trying to thank me for helping her husband to die. "He was so afraid of dying," she said, "and you helped him do that. You did not leave him alone." As she pushed back tears and her voice faded, I again instinctively reached in my shirt pocket. I placed the little black comb in her hand. She clutched it, kept it, and understood.

Fourteen

Snapshot Mentality

It occurs to me as I sit here writing down my thoughts as they come across my current radar screen, that I should share what is on my mind just now. It is almost like these writings are crawling out of the wrinkles that are etched on my aging body, much like the essence of life leaking out through the pores.

After having practiced medicine for over fifty years, and now having been the patient for awhile, I have some reminiscences about it all. I fear that one of the biggest problems I had, and that I see others having now, is the brief nature of our exposure to each other. When one goes to the doctor, the time for sharing is so brief. Decisions are supposed to happen quickly, with such an incomplete database. They can be wrong. The visit is brief by virtue of rules to limit the amount of time for such. It is only a quick "snapshot" in a life that is an epic, a saga, a full-length movie, as it were. One tiny snapshot — not fair to either party in this situation. Often, on the way home, you might think of other "snapshots" the doctor needed to see.

The continuity of things, so necessary if we are to understand each other, is not being factored in to our interactions these days. In the age of fast foods, disposable items, quick fixes of one sort or another, we are losing patience. We are gearing ourselves on such tight schedules that we are "out of synch" with reality. Sometimes we ask questions but don't wait for the answers. Sometimes in our youth, we ask the questions so fast that the older ones of us don't have time to process them. Sometimes the snapshot does not tell the whole story. Even another snapshot brought the next time, maybe a month hence, will disconnect. Memories are not infallible. It becomes a war instead of a warm pleasantry that we look forward to.

I have said all of that to say this. Life is more than a snapshot.

Fifteen

Lesson from Hurricane Hugo

I remember walking about the city of Charleston after Hurricane Hugo, and everywhere I saw the famous old buildings, some dating back to the late 1600s, latticed with scaffolds where workmen were laboring to restore them after the storm. I walked alone with my thoughts. As I looked about and gazed upward, I thought, "These old buildings have stood the test of time, they have stood like principles in the face of the storm. Now they need the scaffolding of young lives to strengthen them and the paint of new brushes to give them a new face — not the demolition ball." Today, amidst storms and changing winds, we need a band of builders, those so visionary that they can build with the strength of new science, together with the cultured and tempered texture of time honored and mellowed art. All of us need to feel the warmth of the embers of the past through lasting and tenured relationships, and to be a part of "the continuity of things." As I continued to walk along, these clear and simple thoughts spilled over to remind me that the essential parts of the practice of medicine that have always been, are now, and will be forever, such as the holding on to the principles, the truths, the classic nature of doing what is right just because it is right, regardless of its political correctness, will stand the tests of future storms. In other words, we would not be tearing down the strong old buildings to replace them with lesser, more modern and likely not as substantial construction. The fears of the future are no match for the strong blood in the veins of dedicated men and women who have a purpose bigger than they are. Such dedication will, as Brandeis said, "fan the embers into flames."

Down by the Creek

Each ripple of the creek across the rocks,
each sound the water and rocks create,
each thought of serenity and the solace of it,
each memory of friends and times past,
each a dividend of an intangible sort.

Never again will this water cross these rocks;
It is on its way to somewhere else — the future.
Never again can we live this day.
But for now, we are in this blessed trance
that contains a freedom
that allows us to appreciate this blessing.
as well as those that have passed us by.

As I sit, mesmerized into stillness
in the movement and energy of this water,
the now of life,
the thought of life passing by,
I am still included in this forceful stream.
It is reminding that there is
a purpose for me.

— *B. Lewis Barnett*

Sixteen

The Dirty Needle

This story touches on the alone times in every person's life. We all have these times, when no matter what, we feel alone. We become frightened, fearing the future. The times are filled with "what ifs." The nighttime seems ominous. The stars don't shine.

Where do we turn? We seem more fragile, more vulnerable.

As I said in the beginning, we are all likely to pass this way. That was certainly true about this particular night. I was sitting in my study about ten-thirty when the phone rang. It was Marty, a fourth year medical student. His voice sounded different than usual. There was an urgency in it, and I waited for the *what next*. "Dr. B (most of the students called me by this moniker), I just stuck my finger with a needle that I was using to draw blood. The patient is an alcoholic; I can't get a good history. I don't know if he has AIDS." "Where are you now?" was my first question. "I am on North 4." I first thought of going into the hospital to be with my friend (and student), but he indicated that he was leaving the hospital to go home, but he felt scared, and since I knew that he lived alone, I suggested that he swing by my house. He seemed to like that idea.

About eleven o'clock there was a light tapping at the front door. At the front door stood a pale and obviously distraught young man. I invited him into the study. We embraced,

43

and tears came. His body literally shook with each sob. I held him until the sobs ceased; then we sat. He was not alone anymore. He related what had transpired. Blood samples had been taken from the patient and from him. Each such incident had to be reported to the folks who handled "Incident Reports." They would follow up on it "in the morning."

In the quietness of the night, away from the hospital, two friends found kindred spirits. There was a lot of silence, there was a sincere prayer, there was a recollection of Psalm 91. We read it, and thinking about this particular night, I just now reread it. It helped.

After awhile, Marty was ready to leave, to go home alone, but not really. He wrote a note a week or so later. It was a short note, only four sentences long. I share two of them with you. "Thank you for helping remind me that while fear can overwhelm us, our faith can conquer fear. After our time together, I again realized that even when leaving by myself I was not alone."

Marty's patient turned out not to have the dreaded disease that he had feared. Now, many years later, he is in great health and practicing in a nearby state. Sharing one's fears with an understanding friend sometimes divides our anxieties in half.

Seventeen

The Way We Remember

Ralph is one of my very favorite cousins, or at least that is the way I remember him when we were growing up. Ralph had three brothers and two sisters living. One other sister had died tragically when she was nine years old. Another brother had died in infancy. His father worked hard as a fixer in the local textile plant, while his mother was kept busy at home taking care of the children.

Every summer Ralph came to spend a couple of weeks in the country with our grandmother, but would split the time around with us cousins and other relatives. I was an only child.

I had not seen Ralph for many years until the other day when we met again at a family reunion. I could hardly believe it when he told me that he and his wife Edith had just celebrated their Golden Wedding Anniversary. So many recollections from our childhood experiences flooded this reunion. These recollections brought back the close feelings I had toward him. He was kind of like the brother I never had. This all came out as we began to swap tales.

The strangest part of it all was how our memories varied, the sharp edges worn off with the passage of time. The same happenings had been like eggs incubating for a long time and only now are bringing forth different hatchlings. In my memory I was thinking how rich he was to have so many brothers and sisters, while I had none. His recollection of how he felt was simply stated. He liked to come visit me because I had more "things" than he did — specifically a bicycle with a speedometer on it! (I had forgotten about the bicycle).

So now here we are, each of us living life on the back nine, reminiscing about how poor and yet how rich we were, all tangled up in childlike thoughts and mellowed memories.

Eighteen

Four Outfits

Most of us are fortunate to have a very few really good and great friends. We have many fair weather ones, but few that we can trust with knowing all there is to know about us and who still like us in spite of that. They are there in sunshine and rain, in the valleys as well as on the mountaintops. Geographic separations do not dim these friendships. Time does not change them.

Let me sketch for you some of my memories of one such trusted friend. This friendship has lasted over six decades now. Victor Greene and I arrived at Furman University in 1943. He was from Chattanooga and I from a much smaller Woodruff, S.C. As he was to say, "Where is that?" The common bond for us was probably that neither came out of a background of affluence. The other bond was that we each knew and felt how fortunate we were to be there. No one in my family had ever had the opportunity to go to college. Vic didn't seem to mind all that. We never talked about the past, just the now, and we enjoyed sharing that "now." He was an aspiring minister, I was an aspiring physician. We had no guarantees that either would make it.

From the very start, we saw in each other something that was worth getting to know better. We understood what it was like living in a world where others seemed to have more "things" than we; this included fancy expensive clothes and automobiles. He had no brothers. I had no brothers. We sort of felt the need for one. That's how it all began. Soon we found out that each of us owned only one suit. If we attended functions often, it was obvious that we wore the same suit every time. We were a mite self-conscious, especially if we dated the same girl with any regularity. Not to be outdone, as my memory serves me, Vic and I decided to pool our wardrobes since we were about the same size. Two suits, two people, but many combinations. His suit, my suit, his coat/my pants, his pants/my coat. You get the idea. This translated into each of us having FOUR different outfits. It made us feel rich.

This kind of understanding and willingness to share whatever we had has lasted for six decades, as I mentioned before. Time has passed by quickly. He became a very prominent and eloquent minister, missionary, and for a time was my personal pastor. But before he was that, he performed our marriage ceremony. He had promised to do that when I ever found the "right" person. Her name was Annalyne. He did a good job; she is still at my side after 44 years. But now to continue the story. I, on the other hand, did become a physician, and for quite a while, Vic's personal physician. My first twenty years I was a country doctor back in my hometown. The next thirty years were spent in academic life at two medical schools, the Medical University of South Carolina (my alma mater) and the University of Virginia at Charlottesville, practicing and teaching.

Once while Vic and Merrily were on furlough from the Philippines for a year, they were staying in Ridgecrest, N.C. Annalyne and I went to visit them there on a very cold January weekend. During this visit Vic said, "Since you like the mountains so much, I know a place that if you saw it you would buy it." With this I said, "Show it to me." We bantered back and forth and found that he was committed to supply a sermon the next day at Spruce Pine, so he would not be able to show it to me the next day. He said, "Get your coat. We can go up there tonight." I thought this strange — no one can see in the dark, and besides, it was January and cold. But in the spirit of our younger adventures together, off we went. Up Highway No. 9 we snaked, over Lakey Gap; then we left the "blacktop" and climbed another two miles to the top of Allison's Ridge. Vic brought the car to a stop out on a point at the end of the road (logging trail would be more descriptive). Before us, on that cold winter night, we could see twinkling stars overhead, and twinkling lights in the valley below. He identified each clump of distant lights one by one. There was Old Fort, Pleasant Gardens, Marion, Forest City, Spindale and Rutherfordton. I was awestruck, if there is such a word.

The next day, Annalyne and I decided to call the number on the sign, and we met Mr. Arthur Hemphill, the owner of the property. He escorted us back up to the top. We quickly made a purchase right then and there. In the ensuing months we cleared a place and hired two mountain carpenters, Clarence Bailey and Joe Pruden, to construct for us a little redwood cabin, like one we saw in a book. The year was 1968. For thirty-four years it has been our place of refuge, as well as for many others, since we have enjoyed sharing it through the years. My feeling is that every doctor needs such a place. Some of you, perhaps a dozen couples, have spent all or part of your honeymoons there. It's a great place to get "really" acquainted.

Through the years, much has changed, but these mountains have not, and the respect that Vic and I have for each other has not. When my father and mother died, it was Vic who I called first. He was eloquent on both occasions and helped us over the rocky times. He had known them both well. He had felt my mother's embraces on many visits. I believe she always considered him with the same love that she always had for me. Rare, I think.

Then, about two years ago, I found myself standing with Vic at the graveside of his beloved wife of fifty years, Merrily. It felt right to be there with him.

It helps me to put pen to paper, or fingertips to the keyboard now, to recall just a few examples of such a wonderful gift, Vic's friendship. May you all be so fortunate to have such a friend. If you do, do not hesitate to tell them just how valuable they are.

Nineteen

At the Women's Social

Three Sundays ago, I was back in my hometown for a family reunion, and is my custom when visiting there, I end my visit by paying tribute to my parents. I go to the cemetery and reverently stand by their graves, and think of times past. On this particular visit, as I stood there, I gazed across the cemetery where so many of my friends, relatives and former patients lay resting. My eyes came upon a tent; underneath it was a yet to be lowered casket. The family had left while the workers "closed" the site. It was my old friend and former patient, Mary Stewart. She had lived to be seventy-nine years old, and as I am told, had spent her last years in the distracted world of Alzheimer's Disease.

But today, as I looked across the cemetery, through the eyes of a country doctor's heart, I remembered the bubbly and vivacious "Miss Mary" who taught my children in the kindergarten as she had done for so many now adults in the community. My memory was flooded with visions of her at younger times. She was such a vivacious and gregarious woman with a buoyant sense of humor, always the life of the party, so to speak. On this day, the vivid story that surfaced had to do with the day that the Presbyterian Women of the Church group in town was having some sort of social gathering. I was not there, of course. I only heard this story from one of the other ladies in attendance who laughed as she recounted it to me. Stories in small towns have an uncanny way of circulating really fast, and usually back to the person who was talked about, often "the doctor."

This story relates, and I now recall its veracity, that Mary was very desirous of having another child, but somehow had not readily conceived. As her doctor, she and I had tried many things, such as diets, thyroid extract, hormones, temperature charts and a modicum of patience. This was in the days before clomid, in vitro fertilization, gift programs, and the like.

At last she was successful, and today was the day when she exuberantly was announcing triumph to her fellow parishioners. As I am told, she said, "Lewis Barnett and I have been trying for a year and a half to get me pregnant!" She announced this with great flourish and brought laughter from the usually prim and proper ladies of the church. Her face turned red as she realized that the remark needed further clarification.

Her delightfully loose and innocent tongue, always openly "telling it like it is," is now silenced. The volume in my memory is, however, turned up to the maximum. This old doctor still remembers and cares very deeply for Mary and her husband, Charles.

Twenty

In Another's Moccasins

A large majority of our patients (maybe most) have something or other that they are not proud of; something about their physical body, their clothing, their habits. Few, if any, are perfect specimens. All have asymmetries, variations, misconceptions of just what "normal" really is. Some feel that they alone possess their perceived imperfections. When made vulnerable by nudity at the hands of medical personnel, they are embarrassed and become more anxious the longer this state is allowed to continue. Our cold hands seem to add to the violation of their privacy and dignity. They anticipate our verdicts and assumptions with fear and apprehension. The moccasin is on their foot, not ours.

Be gentle, be kind, be thoughtful, try to understand and interpret their erratic behavior. They feel vulnerable in the first person. Know that some of their behavior and demeanor is just representative of their best attempt to mount a defense against our intrusion. Most of the time, it is not a personal vendetta against us.

At all points along the way, this shared time should be a time of trust. Do not postpone whatever reassurance you are comfortable to offer. Do it sooner rather than later. We need to do most of our talking, consulting, surmising and sharing with our patients while they are fully clothed so as to make the playing field as level as possible. This would greatly shorten their time on the "unequal" playing field.

Twenty-One

Bigotry and Bias

I have been thinking a lot about our stubborn behavior lately. The more I read and ponder the definitions of bigotry, the more I am convinced that it is present on both sides of the equation. Those holding distinctly different positions on a given subject seem to be equally steadfast, and neither is prone to listen or understand the other. I have long realized that biases and prejudices have kept us from being our most helpful selves. For physicians, accepting our patients as they are and trying to cut through the philosophical differences is difficult for us to do. However, it seems to me that one does not have to sacrifice one's principled core to see the other side of the equation. I believe most of us have a basic inner core of goodness, disguised though it may be. Usually there is "a good side" if we try hard enough to find it. This is not to say that we have to like everyone, or, for that matter, to love their behavior. Even our children try us to the limit sometimes.

Whether one's belief system leans left or right, liberal or conservative, fails to answer the question about understanding and fairness in our actions toward each other. We need to spend less time seeking out differences and more time coming to consensus over just what needs to be done in each instance. Successful outcomes are more likely when consensus, not compliance, is sought. Somehow the word compliance connotes that you insist that the patient does do exactly what you want, even if they do not understand why you are demanding it.

Underlining all of our behaviors, as physician or patient, are the two one-syllabled words: *Right* and *Wrong*. We all need to come to grips with moral, rather than political, correctness. There is a moral high ground. For the sake of all those in need of our help, it is worth seeking. All of this has no monetary dimension. To be rich or poor has nothing to do with the size of our bank accounts, rather the genuineness of our relationships, the love of our fellowmen, and the altruism necessary to rejoice in the other fellows happiness and success. This is hard to do, but even today such remains the balm we need for the aching and anxious souls at our doorsteps. There is so much anguish in our world. If we take the trouble to look underneath the superficial smiles and affected and shallow conversations, we often find a distraught and frightened person. They seem to be overwhelmed at times.

We think that one person cannot make a difference. This is *wrong*. One can make a difference, but not by being afraid or timid. The difference-makers are people just like us, who decide to treat others with respect, even if respect is not given in return. Not gauging our behavior by comparing it to that of others. In assessing "peer pressures," one needs to consider why these pressures should bother us and just how worthy of our attention they really are. Often they are representative of diluted moral values. That brings me to mention the importance of another word, *influence*. One's influence, albeit singular, can stand in the face of such dilute examples rampant in our society today. We can throw our *Pebbles in the Water*. The ripples will take care of themselves.

Twenty-Two

If Physicians Are Artists ...

If indeed physicians are artists as well as scientists of sorts, how then do they create masterpieces? This question has plagued me for a long time, especially since I became involved in the academic world. I wanted so much to try to help young aspiring medical students "to paint masterpieces." By that, I mean, "take diagnosis and treatment to a higher, more personal level; to accomplish the uncommon thing."

Today I sat in church behind a friend. I had heard that he had been undergoing some tests for very low hemoglobin, yet he looked very "pink" to me. As he placed his arm around his wife, I noted that his nail beds were also as pink as mine were. Somehow the person did not match the numbers.

This brought me to the metaphor: Physicians, or at least some of them, are prone to "paint by the numbers." If you do that, you always produce works that are plainly done with brush in hand and little blocks with numbers designating which color to place in certain blocks. That finished product will not be an original. So if we only look at the numbers (results of laboratory tests, studies, etc.), we may never paint the masterpiece. It is only by looking very carefully at the person who has the problem and trying to judge just whether the results look as though they match the clinical appearance of that person, that we enter into a personal assessment. If one depends entirely on laboratory figures and does not allow for error, one robs himself and his patients of the chance to create a personal diagnosis and prescription for treatment. It turns out that one's own brush is clinical judgment, deep personal interest and resolve. Combining all of these with an intellectual interpretation of all available data makes for the masterpiece I envision.

So I return to the question I started with: "If physicians are artists, how then do they create masterpieces?" I say it is by picking up their own personal brush, and with a heightened sense of observation, paint sometimes outside the lines.

(All of these thoughts, of course, came before the sermon started!)

Twenty-Three

Defining Legacy

A legacy is not an object to be physically handed to the next generation. It cannot be wrapped in fancy ribbons. In my mind, legacy is defined as a "process" that is catalyzed by an unselfish relationship between older and younger members of different generations. It is not singular and does not happen in a selfish vacuum. Legacy tends to move past strengths into future, more ambitious potentials.

At best then, legacy is always a "hybrid" — a combination of the seed of the past grown in the fertile soil of a new generation. Is it any wonder that we look at each other, young and old, as if we are some sort of impurity, not being able to feel perfection around us? The feeling that things can always be made better exists.

The leaving of a legacy is a dynamic happening, so subtle and passed so gently that the change becomes seamless. What good would a torch be if there was nowhere to pass it? Where is the value then in this dynamic process? Where is there room for self? Indeed, the moment a torch is passed, someone else, a younger and stronger courier, is waiting to accept it. The legacy contains the strengths of both generations, and its origins are buried in anonymity. To my mind, that is how it should be.

Twenty-Four

Brightly Colored Afghan

Merry Allen was a petite ninety-three-year-old lady. She was a lady in every respect, and when I say petite, I really mean it. She probably measured somewhere between four and five feet tall. Her eyes still had the warmth and sparkle that made it a blessing to be around her.

Her small size had caused her some near death obstetrical experiences. Some babies were stillborn, but she had managed to have one live birth, Evelyn.

Merry's husband was a railroad man and was on the road a lot. His age was just one year more than hers. He had been retired for many years. They had been married for over sixty years. She often laughed, and with a twinkle in her eyes said that she didn't realize that the vows she spoke "in front of God and twenty witnesses" were going to last so long. She also related that on certain days she negotiated her marital relationship by staying in a different room from her husband. Clever, I thought. As long as he was "on the railroad," everything was fine. But as is often the case, retirement brings a new set of problems.

As I said in the beginning, "Miss Merry," as I called her, always had a smile for me. It seemed to fit the spelling of her name. By now though, time had taken its toll and her eyesight was practically gone. That fact makes this story all the more amazing.

One day Evelyn came in with a brightly colored afghan. Pinned to it was a note. I share part of it with you. I am sure she wouldn't mind. "This is given in appreciation and love for the care you have given Mom. She did (all of) the crocheting, and I put the squares together (for her).

"Miss Merry" could not see to assemble the squares, but she crocheted the squares from memory. She knew the pattern. It was a tremendous labor of love. We still cherish it and remember this generous act. She was giving until the end. She always said that doing for others made her feel better, too. I agree.

Do more than exist; live.

Do more than look; observe.

Do more than listen; grasp.

Do more than touch; feel.

Do more than hear; understand.

Do more than think; ponder.

Do more than talk; say something.

— *BLB, 1970*

Twenty-Five

The Rusty Scupper

I had been invited to give the keynote address at the annual meeting of the Georgia Academy of Family Physicians on November 16, 1985. It was held that year in Atlanta, where my daughter Kristen had gone to live post-college. After giving the speech, which she came to hear, by the way, she came up and casually said that her new (boy)friend wanted to take me out to dinner. I said "fine," albeit naively. After relaxing in my hotel room for an hour or so, I went down to the foyer of the hotel where I was staying, fully expecting both of them to pick me up for dinner. It didn't happen that way. Shortly, Jim, the new friend, drove up alone. This twist started all kinds of thoughts; yet I still surmised that we would stop by on the way to the restaurant and get Kristen. That was not to be either. This was to be a stag night.

Jim told me that he had reservations at the *Cork and Cleaver,* a very nice place. Well, sir, we rode and rode until some of the landmarks reappeared, but no *Cork and Cleaver.* We were lost. That was not such a good sign. My new young friend made a quick stop and hurried into a service station to use their pay phone. I had no idea who he was calling. "Could it be Kristen," I mused. Or could he be calling the *Cork and Cleaver?* After all, it was past time for our reservation. Jim was nervous when he returned. That made me nervous.

We started our adventure once more, and pretty soon we pulled in at a different restaurant, the *Rusty Scupper,* whatever that is.

Not having been born yesterday, I was strongly suspicious of this young man's intentions, whereupon I began to formulate a question or so of my own. Prime among my selection was a perfectly appropriate question, that being, "Are you sure?" I was ready.

About halfway through his butterfly shrimp, he stopped eating. He wasn't very hungry. Looking across the table he started, and without inhaling again until he was done, he said, "Dr. Barnett, there is absolutely no doubt in my mind whatsoever that with your permission and Mrs. Barnett's I would like to marry your daughter." Somehow the question I had planned did not seem appropriate at all. The courtship was only nine weeks old! All this time, Kristen was on the phone talking to her mother in Virginia. My wife had gotten the word on what was happening even before I did.

This is the beginning of the story, but as Paul Harvey would say, the rest of the story finds us retired in the Atlanta area, to be near four of our five grandchildren. I think that they were "sure," and I am glad and very proud.

Twenty-Six

Miss Becky's Second Fashion Show

The next day after the memorable dinner at the Rusty Scupper, when Jim asked for my daughter's hand, she came by to take me shopping at Phipps Plaza Mall in Buckhead. It seemed that thousands of Atlantans had the same idea. She and I just ambled our way through the crowd, mostly window shopping. I was just enjoying Kristen's company. She was exuberant today. Wonder why? As we strolled along, and barely out of the corner of my eye, I vaguely caught a glimpse of a lady standing in the door of McGowan's Bridal Shoppe, but somehow nothing registered of familiarity. We passed on by, not having the slightest suspicion that the lady in the doorway would be anyone that I would know. After all, there were millions of people in Atlanta. My plans were to have returned to Charlottesville the day before, but I had extended my stay for a day in view of the major events of last evening.

We walked the full length of this huge mall and back up again. Kristen slowed down and gazed more intently through the window of the bridal shoppe. Her body language was easy to read. We were going in. This same lady was still at the front of the store.

"Dr. Barnett," she screamed loudly, "you were with me the night that Jim died" (her first husband). I did remember her by her first husband's name, Jim Wright. Her name was Becky. We had both been born and raised in the same small town, where I had practiced from 1950 to 1970, with two years out for the Navy. The Wrights were my patients. Indeed, I had made a house call to her home "the night that Jim died." She continued in a lower voice, tears streaming down her cheeks, "You went home and couldn't sleep, so you came back and stayed with me till daylight came."

By this time, the rest of the staff in the store had their eyes focused on us. I was red-faced and speechless. As I am prone to do in such circumstances, I simply gave her a hug. She then looked over at Kristen. The emoting started all over again, because she knew her when she was a little girl.

Becky was the proprietor of a dress shoppe in our hometown during that time. It was called, of course, "Becky's." Annually, or maybe each season, Becky would have a fashion show with refreshments and all. My wife Annalyne and Kristen had been models. As a little girl, Miss Becky had dressed her in fancy dresses! Now she was grown up and about to be engaged to be married.

Becky went on to say that she had felt so bad when she woke up this morning that she didn't feel like coming in to work, but "something" just told her she must get up and go. It might be a special day.

Special it was indeed. I took a seat and relived the past, watching the parade as Kristen and Miss Becky had their own private "fashion show." This time the crowning event was placing a beautiful many-pearl studded hood, veil and all, atop her head. All I had to do was what fathers do, pick up the check!

Twenty-Seven

Dear Mary Waddell

Dear Mary,

This is a long time coming, and now I have waited too late. It is written posthumously. But you see, Mary, I am retired now and I at last have time. The other thing is, I just didn't realize how you felt at the time. You were always there to help me when I was a young doctor working day and night. They called you a nurse's aide, but thinking back, you were more of a doctor's aide, and the patients would even remember you as the one who smoothed the wrinkles in their sheets. After practicing in the small hometown (for both of us) for twenty years, except for a two-year stint in the Navy, I moved away.

I wrestled with the invitation to come back to my Medical School to teach and refused the offer three times. I lost sleep over that, too. But the Professor kept calling, and finally, finally he hit the nerve that touched my heart. Dr. Hiram Curry said, "Lewis, you are up there putting salve on one sore, while the whole state is broken out with an exfoliative dermatitis." Mary, you may not know that last big word I used, but it's pretty bad.

So off we went, family in tow (Annalyne and Lewis and Kristen). You may remember the kids. I used to bring them to the hospital sometimes and they would sit at your desk while I made rounds; then we would be off to make house calls together to the shut-ins. They often brought more cheer than I did.

I say all of that to say this. Just a night or so ago, while thumbing through some of the drawers in my old oak filing cabinet where I have tucked things in no particular order through the years, I ran across a poem, written by hand, your hand, on lined notebook paper. It was the kind of paper that Montag marketed under the logo *Blue Horse*. You had mailed it to us after we left town. As I read it now, thirty-two years later, it brings tears to my eyes. You were so benevolent, even to me. And I, I still feel so undeserving.

If you were here, I would ask your permission to print the words exactly like you said it. Maybe you expressed just what it felt like to be helping, and what your biased opinions were of a doctor just doing the best he knew how. I did not know you were watching so closely, but after all, you were there and I guess I didn't realize that you were such a detective.

So, Mary, thank you, from the bottom of my heart. Forgive me for waiting so long, and for sharing your literary work with everybody.

Her Poem

To the finest doctor I know,
you never did put on a big show.
You always treated patients day to day,
even if they were not able to pay.

Our friendship began when I walked in the hospital door;
that was sixteen years ago and more.
We talked with each other and I made rounds with you,
and from that day on I always helped with your deliveries too.

After you made your rounds each day,
you would turn around and say,
"If you need me tonight, just dial the phone
because I will be at home.

Underneath that nice new suit,
your heart always beat strong,
always full of love and loyalty.
What's more, you always proved it, too.

Dr. Barnett, you were always professional and nice, too.
You had more friends than any doctor galore,
and you were always near
when an emergency came to our hospital door.

You helped my husband when he was sick and in doubt,
but today, Dr. Barnett, we are so happy we could shout.
If we can ever do anything for you, just let us know in a hurry.
Just dial Woodruff Hospital and ask for old Mary.

You have lots of papers
about your family tree,
but, Dr. Barnett, you could always make it
with or without a degree.

I know you are happy with your work today,
and, Dr. Barnett, don't you ever forget to pray.
Marvin and I are always discussing your work and you
and about the wonderful things you did for us, too.

— *Mary Waddell, 1970*

Thank you, thank you, Mary. I will tell everybody not to wait as long as I did to thank somebody who has made a real difference in this world.

— BLB

Twenty-Eight

Special Delivery

As some of you know, I have just observed (I won't say celebrated) my seventy-sixth birthday. This story is about one of the happenings that day. The doorbell rang with its cheery chime. I got up from my desk and answered the door. There stood our mail lady with package in hand. I accepted it and thanked her. Not often, at least in my experience, are deliveries brought to your door and personally put into your hands, but that is what happened on this particular day.

I noticed that the package was from two of my former patients from Charlottesville, Helen* and Arthur. They are my friends as well as former patients. Upon my retirement, my wife and I moved away from Charlottesville and relocated near our daughter, son-in-law and four of our five grandchildren in the Atlanta area. Our address since February of 2000 has been Kennesaw, Georgia.

I hastened to open up the package. As I did, the aroma of fresh-baked bread gave the secret away. You see, Arthur is a baker of bread extraordinaire. This is but one of his many talents. On previous birthdays Helen and Arthur had delivered a loaf of his signature bread to our home in person. Now it is not possible to do so since we live 560 miles apart.

I stared at the wrapping and was shocked when I saw that the postage to ship this loaf was $21.15. "Incredible," I said, but then I thought, "Incredible friends." It was a gift prepared by hand, just for me. The amount of postage was just a barometer of a genuine friendship to be cherished now, perhaps more than ever before. The bread had been carefully wrapped in foil and shipped for overnight delivery and was still fresh. As I peeled back the silvery wrap, the happy thoughts of the moment turned to more pensive thoughts of days gone by. I sliced into it and savored the aroma, which brought back so many memories of many times when we had faced problems together.

Not a crumb was wasted. Thanks, Helen and Arthur. Who else would have thought of such?

(*This piece was written on the afternoon of August 11, 2002. Arthur called to say that Helen died of a massive stroke the next morning, August 12th. Age 89. One of a kind, she was.)

Unsung Heroes

Getting the marble out of the quarry is the tough part of creating a masterpiece. Those who do this are always the unsung heroes of the artistic worlds. The "behind the scenes" folks, who many believe their work to be unimportant, are all a necessary part of the process. No honest labor is without purpose and meaning. It is a vital part of any finished product.

Twenty-Nine

What Christ Means in My Daily Work

The following thoughts were scribbled with pencil, in the middle of the night, in the dark, during the wakeful time as I waited for sleep to come during the busy days of general practice. The date was in the 1960s and the place was Woodruff, South Carolina. I was thirty- four years old. I share this with you now (2002) because I still hold to these beliefs.

A Partner — when I feel alone
A Strength — when weakness creeps over me
A Companion — when everything seems unfriendly
A Wisdom — when I am dumb
A Hope — when human skeptics give up
A Friend — when I least deserve one
A Humility — when I am prone to feel overly important
A Significance — when I am impotent
An Understanding — when someone needs to be understood
An Extra — when the usual is not sufficient
A Warmth — when the climate of my soul is cold
A Silence — when everything else is too loud
A Radiance — when all I can see is darkness
A Solution — when my meager knowledge runs out
A Profit — even if nobody pays.

— *BLB, 1960*

Thirty

I'm Coming

There are times in every doctor's life when he or she listens to a patient's tortuous story and draws a complete blank. It is a very lonesome feeling, knowing that the person looks to us for answers. When a patient looks us in the eye and expects us to know more than we do know, it places us in an uncomfortable position. Among other things, it gives us a tremendous stimulus to dig deeper, to hit the books, to seek a consultation, or to simply just listen a little while longer hoping that the "light will come on."

I remember one night when the phone rang after I had gone to bed. I answered it almost before I had fully awakened. The voice on the other end of the phone sounded distraught and babbled a galaxy of disjointed symptoms, with the admonition to come quickly. When I hung up, I thought to myself that I had never heard of such a disease. It was one of those moments when you wondered just what the professors had and had not taught you in medical school. As I sleepily put on my clothes, stumbling in the dark to get each leg to go down the right way, I remembered the last words I had said before I hung up. "I'm coming, I'm coming. Leave the light on."

As I made my way down Cross Anchor Road toward the house I was to find in the middle of a bunch of trees with fields all around, my blank mind kept playing the tape of the incongruous conversation over and over. It was not until I walked up the three or four steps and went into the door that was being held open by a frightened wife that I began to put things together. It was only after I sat down by the bedside, smelled the odors that were released when the quilts were thrown back, saw the expression on the fellow's face, felt his hot skin, and asked him just how he felt that the pieces of the puzzle fell into place.

On my way home, with the peace one gets when things go well, I replayed my last words before hanging up the phone. "I'm coming. I'm coming."

In this case that made all the difference.

Thirty-One

Wonder Why That Is?

You will have to think very hard to understand that the elements of this true story really happened, but I promise you it did happen. It involves a rather quaint woman who carved for herself a very special place in my practice. On the first visit to see me as her new physician, she brought a very large piece of stiff parchment, measuring about twelve inches square. On it, sectioned off into compartments were neatly printed lists of her complaints diligently categorized. As I looked at her, dressed in an unusually long dress which spoke to a style of earlier days, a collection of beads from various parts of the world, a kind of vintage hat that sat cocked to one side of the head, and uniquely shaped small spectacles — and then looked back at the parchment, I prayed for patience and an uncommon portion of wisdom. She had registered using three surnames, a couple of family ancestors' names, as well as a maiden name and a married name. She had been divorced for many years and was living alone. She owned a house in Charlottesville, Virginia, and also one in Little Rock, Arkansas. Her basic roots were in Arkansas.

For starters, we made an agreement that I would start by taking one "compartment" at a time, letting her prioritize them as to importance or urgency. I handled the parchment very carefully, treating it much like the Holy Grail. She seemed to appreciate that.

Over time and many visits later we addressed all of the symptoms in her self-concocted syndromic blocks. We had come to appreciate one another and were now friends — for life. One day she announced that she needed to go back to Little Rock for awhile, maybe permanently. She promised to come back to see me from time to time. The look from her earnest eyes caused me to believe that she really would.

After about a year, I noticed her name on my 3x5 inch card that my secretary always gave me with names of patients for that day. Beside her name were the two words, "check up." When I walked into the room where she was, she stood up, arms outstretched, and we embraced and acted like long lost friends reunited. An exotic but very different perfume proved to be enough for both of us, with some left over for a room on either side of number six.

It turns out that she had made the journey from Little Rock alone, driving her trusty little Dodge Colt car, using a lot of back roads. That was quite a feat since she was not the healthiest or the youngest woman on the roads. I was humbled by the fact that she took the risks involved for such a trip.

After accomplishing the check-up, all the while listening to a banter of vintage complaints that had become old friends by now, as well as this year's new and fresh ones, we sat together as I reviewed the parchment. I had kept it archived in true parchment fashion, folded into quarters and pressed between the pages of her chart. There was an end to her chatty demeanor. It was quiet. After a period of silence, she said, "I always feel better after I have seen you. I wonder why that is?" I was touched. I presided over a period of silence and finally said, "I don't know. I wonder why that is, too." She continued, "You touch my body where it hurts, physically. You know me. You seem to appreciate my needs. You listen."

Such a simple analysis: I wonder why that is, that such basic and innocent exchanges between trusting friends can possess such strong magnetism and connection? But there we sat, really deep down inside knowing "why that is." The little Dodge Colt had joined the project and brought her safely to this place today. The cocky hat had made the trip, too.

Thirty-Two

Who Is in There?

During the years of 1949-50 I served my internship at the Episcopal Hospital at the corner of Front Street and Lehigh Avenue in northeast Philadelphia. It was in a blue-collar neighborhood; the streets were lined with row houses. As interns we rarely ever "got off the reservation." When we did, the folks along the streets were friendly to us because we usually wore the white uniforms with the barber-necked collars. These were the years when you could walk the streets safely, but not any more. My favorite restaurant was Joe's Place. He served the best Italian seasoned hamburger steak. Since our stipend was zero, that's all I could afford and that very rarely. The Episcopal Hospital was a century-old collection of stone buildings connected by underground tunnels. In the middle of this complex of buildings stood a chapel. It was unusual in that the back half was not equipped with pews. Patients who were bedfast were brought down in the elevators and wheeled in to fill the blank spaces.

This story took place as I was walking past the opening into the chapel. I was sleep deprived from a busy night in the Accident Ward, so I was heading up to my little room where we had a cot to catch a few winks. It was Christmas Eve. I was suddenly aware of a tug on the side of my pants. I looked down and there, looking up at me, was a cherubic little Italian lad with bright eyes and a quizzical countenance. He asked, "Doctor, who is in there?" pointing to what seemed to be an empty chapel. I answered, "Nobody." I walked on. He followed behind and tugged again. He asked the same question over. My answer was the same. By this time, I turned to face him and bent over to catch him at eye level. He looked me straight in the eye and said, "I think God is in there. It sure looks like His house."

"You are right," I admitted. "You are right."

The next day was Christmas and I was on call again. This was a special Christmas. I had been reminded by a little guy that indeed, everywhere I walked I was not alone.

Thirty-Three

Put Them Through, Dora

Busy doctors have many demands on their time. That surely is one of the more redundant statements that could be made in modern times. I started out my practice as a single man; therefore I developed habits that totally consumed my days and nights caring for my patients. I was completely at their beck and call. I never learned how to say "no."

As the months passed, I became a married man. The old habits had to be altered, but how? My world now suddenly held more obligations and expectations from new directions. Medicine had become a jealous mistress, hard for my wife, or any doctor's wife, to understand or appreciate. Being torn in many directions demands an intricate balancing. There is no if, or but, or maybe about it. This needs attention.

Soon our first child, son Lewis III, arrived; then about nineteen months later along came daughter Kristen. More responsibilities, more dimensions to my existence came, and the practice grew and grew and grew. The need for broader, stronger shoulders was evident. There can be no singular existence; life now includes many, many others; the most important ones are your wife and children. I was not the only one doing a balancing act. My dear wife had to balance her time. Now she had three "babies," including me! She faithfully brought lunch to the office in the proverbial brown bag. She and I were both balancing.

One wonders where the children were in all of this. They had not yet learned the balancing act. They only knew and felt that they often needed Daddy. No argument there; indeed they did. I feel that after over forty-three years, they still do.

Without the help of a very special person, all of this might not have happened. Her name is Dora. She was my very dependable, "extra member of the family." You see, Dora "ran" my office, answered the telephone, was my receptionist, bookkeeper, and sometimes nurse. She had direct contact with the outside world while I had my nose buried in the small examination rooms down the hall. She and I worked out a deal, a very important one as it turns out. Simple, but huge! The deal was that whenever either of the children called and asked for Daddy, she would put them straight through to me, no matter what, even if she had to hold the phone for me. Often both of my hands were tied up!! Many "crises" and problems were handled this way. They both felt that they were top priority. Daddy was there for them. Dora still remembers, I still remember, and both Lewis and Kristen still remember. They are now parents (with cell phones yet!).

Thanks, Dora.

Life does not hold still.

Sometimes one must click
the shutter at the crucial moment.

As Eudora Welty did so well,

she felt the need to hold

transient life in words.

So do I.

Thirty-Four

E Pluribus Unum

Over the years Annalyne and I have received many wedding invitations, but this one was different. On the outside it looked similar to all of the others, but upon opening it there was a small, perhaps three by three inches, piece of paper. One edge was torn so that you could tell that it had been part of a larger piece. On it was written, "Just a note to let you know that I finally made it to the "big" step. If it hadn't been for you and, of course, God's help — I might not be here." It was signed, Anita.

What Anita was alluding to was something I am sure she didn't remember first hand but had been told about. It happened the day she was born. When I finally was able to deliver her, she was limp and breathless. She required an unusually long (it seemed) resuscitation effort. All present, including her father, felt that saving her was hopeless. One last effort with mouth-to-mouth resuscitation brought forth a gasping breath, and a new life was meant to be.

Now she is getting married. I appreciate the little note tucked in this wedding invitation.

Thirty-Five

Touching a Toe

I have kept a one-page handwritten letter on brown University of Virginia stationery dated 2/16/88 in my files through the years. This is being written fourteen years later. This letter is from George who was a second year medical student at the time that he wrote it. Until he reminded me in this letter, I had dismissed the incident he mentions because it seemed so insignificant.

You see, George was a very athletic fellow who loved to play soccer. In a pick-up game a year before (1987) he had sustained a severe fracture of his right femur. He had been placed in a cast up to his waist. He was flat on his back

Since he was a popular medical student, he was inundated with visits from classmates and other friends. Hospitals are really no place to rest and have peace. I hesitated to add even one more visitor to the crowd, but after all, he was a student of mine, and I cared about him. So I went up to his room, thinking that if he were asleep I would not wake him up. As I walked softly and quietly into his room, I noticed that his eyes were shut, so I started backing toward the door. Suddenly, he grimaced and opened his eyes. His eyes caught mine and he motioned for me to come nearer without uttering a sound.

As I approached the bedside, I could see the full extent of his cast. He could not move his right leg. Only the end of his great toe was exposed. George could not feel it or reach it. I touched it and casually noted aloud that the color was pink so the circulation was good. That was that.

Getting back to the letter which was sent a year or so later, in it he shares, "I especially remember the healing touch you brought to my toe (which seemed a very big issue to me at the time) and how much it meant to me for someone to understand."

Such a small thing, I thought, but not small to George.

Coupling

One of the dangers of aging is stagnation.

One of the dangers of being young is instability.

With aging comes tested experience.

With being young one embraces change.

Experience coupled with change

gives stability to new ideas.

— BLB, 1992

Thirty-Six

I Ran Away

Our next door neighbors were the Tabors. We were good friends. One evening the phone rang and it was Sylvia. She pleaded for me to come quick. I went straightaway, and when I got there Harvey was sitting dazed in his recliner. He stared at me as though I were a perfect stranger. After a few moments of silence, he said, "Who are you? I don't know you." This went on for a few minutes, and finally his countenance changed and his eyes brightened up as he said, "Hello, Lewis, what are you doing here?"

This was the first of many Transient Ischemic Attacks. Over time, the neurologic episodes became more severe. Harvey was admitted to the small hospital in my town for observation. I had made arrangements for him to be transferred to the much larger hospital twenty-five miles distant. As we waited for the transportation to arrive, his wife was with him in the last room on the right side of the corridor. I was sitting at the nurse's desk. Suddenly I heard screams coming from that direction. It was Sylvia running up the hall yelling and sobbing so that everyone in the little hospital could hear. Harvey had abruptly ceased to breathe. He was dead. We could not resuscitate him. The autopsy revealed many vascular changes, some abnormalities of long-standing.

We grieved together, Sylvia and I, and after six months I realized that she was not doing any better with her loss. On a visit to the office, she began to recount that day. She said that she had been haunted with the dream in which she was screaming, "I ran. I ran away. I abandoned him. I left him." I answered by saying, "No, Sylvia, you have it all wrong. You didn't run AWAY. You *ran* FOR HELP." The small word change after the word ran made all the difference. Forever after that, she could hold her head up, and in her heart she knew that she ran for help indeed.

Thirty-Seven

You Can't Help Me

On any given day you might have a patient to present with a defensive prologue to start the visit. It happened to me many times. Margaret comes to mind as a good, or bad, example. She was a rather stern and stoic German lady, the wife of one of my colleagues. Her first comment to me was, "You can't help me, Doctor. I wouldn't be here if my husband (a doctor himself) had not arranged for it. I have been to many doctors. None have helped. They all gave up on me."

Well, talk about starting at the bottom! I gripped my armchair tight, breathed deeply, and began with, "If you don't mind, just tell me what you think is the biggest problem." She began by relating that she had not had a normal elimination for twenty-nine years. She could not go anywhere socially, because it took her all morning to take care of that problem. First she tried instilling enemas, holding them in while she made the beds, then maybe had to repeat several times during the morning. She related that her mother lived in Germany and she could not visit her because of "this terrible problem."

As I listened her out, I kept thinking about the time frame of the problem (a good thing to do). My next comment, "Tell me what happened twenty-nine years ago." As it turns out, she was married and got pregnant on the honeymoon, which led to a very, very difficult labor that produced an eleven-pound baby. To add to this saga, nine months later she gave birth to another oversized daughter. The recuperation was less than pleasant. She had extreme lacerations and scarring in the organs of reproduction and nearby structures. So we did have the significant piece of history. The gastroenterologists she had seen in the past apparently didn't ask that question and maybe didn't get this bit of vital information.

Now that I had a starting place, and she had started with her "You Can't," I made some rather bold statements to counter hers. Mine began, "First, I will say that you have overwhelmed many of the doctors who tried to help you. I will not let you overwhelm me. Many efforts have failed on the first try and you have discarded them. I will try one thing and if it doesn't work, I will keep trying until something does work. Others have shut the door on you, hoping you would never come back. I will not shut my door. If it shuts, you will be the one to do it. Others and even you may not have given time for the remedies to work. I will give them time. I will be patient with you if you will be patient with me."

She sat stunned. Her blustering entrance behavior was gone. She doubted, and well she should, but she did not leave the room in anger.

Many weeks went by as we tried one regime after another. According to her later comments, she almost gave up on herself and me many times, but somehow she decided to keep trying. Several months went by. She called to tell me what had happened. She had almost given up when she had an abnormally large elimination, "Like having a BABY!" Aha, a baby too big. Now it is done. She has a ticket to Germany to see her dear mother, whom she hasn't seen for many, many years.

Thirty-Eight

If You Are So Inclined

The date was January 29, 1948. I was a junior medical student at the Medical University of South Carolina in Charleston, and our class was assembled in the amphitheater waiting for a lecture on surgery. On this particular day the lecturer was scheduled to be Dr. Horace G. Smithy. The hushed atmosphere in the classroom was different this day. Rumors had been going around for several days that Betty Lee Woolridge, a frail 21-year-old woman had been flown down from her home in Canton, Ohio. It was known that she was willing to be the first human ever to allow a surgeon (Dr. Smithy) to perform a commissurotomy on her stenotic (scarred) mitral valve. We had known that Dr. Smithy had experimented with 120 dogs, but never had he performed this surgery on a human being. For that matter, neither had anyone else. His interest was very personal in that he himself had a stenotic aortic valve. He was fighting the clock with his own life. He was trying to train a younger surgeon to do this operation on himself. According to the rumors, this was the day of the operation. We really did not expect him to lecture to a bunch of third year students on such a momentous occasion. What was to follow has left a graphic memory of that day.

The hush deepened as Dr. Smithy entered the room. He stood in silence, then turned to the blackboard, picked up a piece of chalk, and printed in bold letters, SURGERY OF THE HEART. After carefully and deliberately underlining those words, he laid his chalk down, looked up at us, and after a long period of silence, he spoke, "Those of you who are so inclined, PRAY." After this, he left the room in dead silence. We sat there in awe, knowing that he was walking across the street to become a part of the history of Cardiac Surgery. In those early days, there were no heart-lung machines. The procedure was done on the beating heart, injected with local anesthetic to control the erratic rhythm. The technique involved a purse-string suture and a tiny blade called a valvulotome used blindly just feeling for the diseased valve.

Betty Lee Woolridge survived this procedure. Her color and vigor returned to near normal.

On October 28, 1948, when I was a senior, Dr. Smithy died at 5:30 a.m. before any younger surgeon could muster the courage to operate on him. He was only 34 years old. Within weeks of his death Betty Lee Woolridge died. Her attachment to and love for Dr. Smithy was so great. Her heart was broken. Grief proved to be too much. The bond between them carried with it a very high price.

Thirty-Nine

Breast Lump

As was my custom, I entered the room where Eudora was sitting, and after the usual pleasantries, I asked, "So what brings you here today?" I had noticed that my pocket card of patients to be seen had the notation "breast lump" by her name. Sure enough, that is what she said.

I began my search for the breast lump, but try as I might, I could not discern a lump in either breast. She seemed almost disappointed that I had failed to find "it." At that point, I noticed tears in her eyes. Knowing that I had not found a lump, but that I had touched a much more sensitive and personal spot, I waited in silence, holding her hand in mine. The tears came in abundance.

The next few minutes brought an unraveling of the real reason she came today. Twenty years ago on this very day, her husband had gone fishing and suffered a fatal attack while out in his favorite boat. Her brother was dying of cancer, her husband's aunt was also dying. All of these memories were accentuated by other sad times in her life. She had lost a teenage son by suicide. She needed to unload these burdens. She needed not to carry them home. She needed a companion now.

The moral of this story is that the ticket for a visit with the doctor is not always where the real problem is to be found. There was no lump in the breast, but there was a mountain that she needed someone to help her climb today.

Sometimes, in the moments of silence, the unexpected happens. We do not always know what anniversaries we are attending.

Forty

I Can See

There are many stories surrounding the remarkable life of Rita Faye. I believe they each touch a different chord. That is why I want to share each fascinating experience. Just the other night during supper the phone rang. I am sure that you get the message that the phone really does know when I sit down to the dinner table! This time a voice that I had never heard on the phone before was very loud and clear. "Dr. Barnett, this is Rita Faye. You may not remember me."

I quickly blurted out, "Oh, yes, I do remember you. I delivered you. You weighed one pound and four ounces when you were born (567 grams)."

She continued, "I have been trying to find you. Now I have finally found you. I will soon be thirty-six years old. Her birth date flashed in my memory. She was born on September 28, 1958. Excuse me for interrupting. She went on, "I have a fourteen-year-old son and an eight-year-old daughter. *My memory of having held her in my right hand, her arms and legs not hanging over the edges of my palm, almost blocked out her conversation. How tiny her uterus and ovaries must have been. We fed her with an eye dropper and hypodermoclysis, using tiny 2x2 gauze pads for diapers. She was discharged on Christmas Eve. The nurses tied a huge red ribbon around her before they handed her to her mother.*

Rita interrupted my thoughts to say, "I remember being in the incubator. They all say I couldn't possibly remember that, but I do." This I found hard to believe, too, but then she said she remembered the red bow and lots of presents. Such stories are now indelibly emblazoned on her brain, so let's just leave them alone.

Now to get to the main reason she called. It was to tell me that she had recently had an operation on her eyes. She had cataracts and, "Now I can really see," she gleefully exclaimed. I had feared that her legal blindness may have been due to retrolental fibroplasia, although I had never ordered that she get more than one liter of oxygen. She stated joyfully with a lilt in her voice, "I just knew you would want to know. Mama always told me that you worried about my eyes. Would you send me a picture, I want to see how you look." *I sent her the only recent one I had, knowing full well that it would probably burst her illusions.*

This story covers thirty-six years. Sometimes it takes time and patience to see how some decisions play out in life. The lilt in Rita's voice was payment enough for the long wait. The fact that she "knew" I would want to "know" was enough in itself to make the doctor feel better.

{All of this is even more amazing as I recollect that there were no neonatologists then and no newborn intensive care units or nurses. The hospital was a small fifty-bed facility in South Carolina.}

A Little Word, Kaizen

One of the most important little words that I have come to appreciate is the word Kaizen. My understanding is that this little word is Japanese in its common usage. I am told that in English, it is translated: tiny, continuous improvements that lead to more successful outcomes. Putting tiny together with continuous and improvements seems to hold the secret of making a difference, albeit subtle, in our daily lives. This, to me, is another one of those tiny pebbles thrown into the smooth, glassy waters around us to create ever so gently those concentric rings of influence that spread slowly but surely to benefit others. The strange part of this whole story is that we may never see where this influence finally touches its intended and needed space. Kaizen — tiny, continuous improvements that lead to more successful outcomes — we do not have to know whose lives they touch.

Forty-One

Dean of Women

Kate is a very independent, strong-willed former school teacher and once the Dean of Women at a teacher's college. For so long, she has really been *in charge*. She has been a power-packed human dynamo. Her vital statistics include the fact that her husband Gus had a long downward spiral for most of their married life. He finally succumbed to the genetic disease, muscular dystrophy. She had to be the bread winner and caretaker, too. She herself has had several heart attacks, two cancers (breast and colon), and hypertension that is hardly measurable. All of this she has battled.

She has only one child, a daughter, who never married for fear of passing on the genetic problem. She had also seen two of her uncles die of complications of muscular dystrophy, too. This was heavy baggage for her. She had felt left out because her mother did not have much time for her. She also was angry with her father for having the bad gene and therefore could not sympathize with him. The emotions fought in the cauldron of reality.

Despite her strong will and defensive behavior through the years, it is different now. She is an octogenarian. Finally, her daughter has had all she can take from the years of cool dominance she has felt. She packed her belongings and moved out west, some two thousand miles away from her mother, leaving her to fend for herself. Among other things, she took along her anger and bitterness.

Now Kate is losing those characteristics of strength and the ability to "handle things herself" that so many have admired. In desperation and anger she is blasting everyone who tries to help her. She cuts down the doctors one by one. She literally bites the hands that feed her. Why do humans seem to turn against those who care the most?

It is hard. How can we manage this syndrome that I have come to call *Anger At Large?* Surely she can't hate us THAT much. Surely we do not deserve her vitriolic outbursts. How can we keep our sense of mission in the face of such wild and volcanic antagonism and criticism? How can we give her peace?

I sit. I think. I try again. I know very well that all of my efforts are always at risk of being misunderstood. My job is to fight against the human temptation to *write her off, to give up.* Granted, it takes uncommon love in its purest form to handle her problems. Rightly she says, "You just don't know!" It takes real courage to stick with these folks, to hang in there, to be there, to assure them at the very least they do not face the future alone. Let them know that the door is open, that you will not shut it no matter what, even if they themselves slam it in your face.

Kate's *former* self would have appreciated our efforts. I know she needs a friend more than she ever has. "Forgive her," I tell myself. She needs to make friends with herself, but she doesn't want to do that, because she does not even like the person she has become.

Forty-Two

Blue Concrete

Ruth is a senior citizen as our generation is now labeled. She is a veritable storehouse for memories. Some are good but some are bad. We sometimes find it easier to remember the bad things than it is to remember the good. She suffers now from severe osteoporosis, made more severe because of her bitterness toward her former doctor. You see, she is mad because he did not prescribe estrogens and all of the other remedies she has read about. She has let the anger literally rob her of any pleasure in life. She never smiles anymore. She has reluctantly signed on with a new young doctor. He sincerely wishes that he could help in some way. I know he cares because he has shared her case with me. Even though we live on opposite sides of the country, we have shared her in our thoughts by way of the telephone. What we share in common is simple. He cares and I care. The worst of Ruth's problem was the bitterness, worn so close to the surface that no one wanted to be around her. It was compounded by this self-imposed exile with its loneliness. The first visits with her new doctor were not filled with positive thoughts.

We tried to understand her difficulty with accepting sincere efforts on her behalf. The truth was, she did not think anyone would help her, and this alone was discouraging for the doctor. As time went on, Ruth did open up gradually, sharing her biography in bits and pieces. She had worked for one of the local industries in town for twenty-nine "of the best years of her life." As she shared, the doctor began to see more and more about her that he liked and that he admired. The chemistry between them was building. He began to look forward to her visits, instead of dreading them. Her biography began to reveal bigger chinks of time. Flashbacks gave the doctor a clearer image of the younger Ruth — vital, certainly much taller. Now she needed desperately to shed from her weakened shoulders the burden of so much resentment. Some of the newer medicines, according to her, just may be helping "a little," but still there were no smiles.

As an important aside to Ruth's story, the plant where she had given "twenty-nine of the best years of her life" was being demolished to make way for "progress." To her, this was just a sign of it "being in the way" and of no more use. To look upon the pile of debris saddened her. One day her doctor went by the site. He stopped the car, got out and went over to the rubble and picked up a piece of stucco that showed that it had absorbed many coats of different colors of paint over the years. The most recent one was blue. He tucked what some would call rubble in his pocket and drove away to his office where he placed it in his desk drawer.

On Ruth's next visit, at an appropriate moment, he opened the drawer and lifted the blue piece of concrete out and handed it tenderly to Ruth with the comment, "You spent a lot of years at this plant, I think you deserve a piece of it." The blue concrete was suddenly transformed from rubble into a semi-precious stone. You would have thought that it was a giant sapphire. At last, Ruth smiled bigger than she had in years. The calcium she needed in her bones became secondary to the "calcium" she had found for her soul. It represented a part of her life and revealed the kind of caring doctor who knew that all therapies do not come from the pharmacy.

Forty-Three

Splendor Intensified

I am sitting on the deck of my mountain cabin. Some call it *High Rock,* I call it *Distant Hills.* No matter what you call it, there is an aura about this place.

It is autumn. Leaves, some like birds, others like butter-flies, are taking flight today. They are lifted by unseen breezes. It is so quiet you can hear their journeying through space. The sun is casting its rising shadows on the coves. There is an overwhelming backdrop of bursting colors — reds, yellows, some evergreens still — nature's show at its best.

With many eyes, the eyes of family and friends who are not even here with me today, I look at this majestic, God-given, intricately decorated scene. Yes, and with the efforts I conjure up to enjoy it all through the many missing eyes of friends who have been here with me on other days, who mean so much to me still, the colors seem to turn up their intensity. The profusion envelopes me. Suddenly I am not alone. It is as if they are here.

A tiny, tiny real bird soars high over all of this, giving life to this colorful spectacle and adding another significant dimension.

The memories of times past when others have sat here with me stir my soul to realize what blessings they are. Out of all this, I have found why this spot is hallowed ground for me. Without the sharing of all this with those I love and cherish, it would not have been the same. Those of you who have been here with me understand what I am trying to express. Those of you who have not will just have to try to.

Forty-Four

In Search of Flander's Ointment

One day I was back in my hometown where I had practiced for twenty years. I was there primarily to visit my ninety-year-old mother who lived in the small hospital there. Her elderly caretaker had sent me to the drug store in search of Flander's Buttocks Ointment, a local wonder concoction purported to ward off bed sores. It must work, for my mother had never had one. It must be the balsam in it, I surmised.

While going down the aisle where all of the salves were lined along the shelves, I was surprised by a young woman approaching me from behind. She began to speak to me in a most familiar fashion. "You don't remember me, but you delivered me. I'm Marguerite's daughter." With that introduction, all kinds of bells started ringing. I said, "Is Rita Faye your sister?" She replied, "Yes, sir." My next question was, "How is she?" (You see, she weighed one pound and four ounces when I delivered her back in September of 1958.) The answer came, "Oh, she's fine. She has two children now, a boy and a girl. She got married, had a boy, then divorced, then remarried the same man and had a girl. They are doing fine."

So, on the hunt for Flander's Ointment, in the back aisle of the local drug store, I chanced upon a precious part of my past. I had held Rita Faye in one hand. Her arms and legs did not hang off the edges of my palm, and now her progeny are headed toward normal lives and yet another generation. It makes one wonder why it is so hard to believe in miracles.

By the way, I found the Flander's Buttocks Ointment, too.

Forty-Five

Human Splint

When a bone is fractured and the fragments are out of place, the two ragged edges are not in apposition (fitting). Our first order of business is to gently try to straighten them and place a plaster splint to make the situation less painful, more comfortable, to make it more stable. This story starts as an orthopedic problem, and we can understand the problem and its solution.

When a life is "fractured," fragmented, and relationships have ragged edges and understanding of the problem is not so simple, the injured person cries out for solution. Sometimes you can be a "human splint" for such a "fractured" life. Gently and carefully listening and feeling the displacement of the fragments. I say gently, and carefully, because a splint or cast that is applied too tight can cut off normal circulation and can prevent healing. And just as a plaster cast is beneficial for a time, if left too long this allows the muscles to atrophy (wither) and become weakened.

Knowing when to remove the splint or cast is crucial. The taking off is as vital as the putting on. Our desire to help, if overdone or prolonged, can satisfy our own "need" to be needed, but in the process the overzealous nature of some tends to weaken the person we are trying to help.

One of the most blessed opportunities we have is to be a human splint for a fractured life. One of the most essential parts of extending the helping hand is the inner knowledge of when to withdraw it and let the person stand alone, exhibiting the effort to strengthen their own muscles — becoming less needful of us.

Like so many reactions in the Chemistry laboratory, there must be a catalyst. Like so many end results, the catalyst is never evident in the finished product. It was necessary for the catalyst to be involved to bring about the result, but not necessary to be heralded in the end. So it is with our kind deeds, our understanding, our wisdom, and our appropriate place in another's life.

Forty-Six

Peaks and Valleys

June 2, 1978 was a momentous day for me. My wife and our two children, as well as my aging parents, were all gathered together in one place. This in itself was a rare occasion, but today was very special. My Alma Mater, Furman University, was awarding me the honorary Doctor of Laws degree. In addition, I was also to give the commencement address. Dr. John Johns, Furman's president, had admonished me to be brief. Since it was very hot, and my parents were in the audience, I was glad to oblige. As I recall, the talk lasted about sixteen minutes.

The pomp and circumstance of the occasion was a very emotional time for a fellow who never in a million years would have expected to be here for such. It had a surreal dimension to it. They must have the wrong fellow. Being center-stage and under the hot spotlights, I could feel the sweat running down my back under the thick black robe. Well, wrong fellow or not, I was here.

After we had attended the reception by the lake and had said good-bye to faculty, family and friends, we packed up and started the 350-mile trip back to Charlottesville. As I said, it was a blistering hot day in June and we were enjoying the air-conditioned car, while we reminisced over what had just transpired.

Suddenly, between Danville and Lynchburg, the car lurched to the side as the right back tire exploded. We came to an abrupt halt and got out to survey the situation. We had come to a leaning stop on the side of the road where there was just not much, if any, shoulder. After a search of the trunk, I assembled the car jack, *little* spare tire and lug wrench. Then began the ordeal. First, there was no level ground, the car was tilted, there was no place for me to have a level spot to squat. The lugs were stripped and the wrench could not engage them properly. My wife climbed down in the ditch behind me to pick the ticks off of my sweaty back. It seems we had invaded their territory. The earlier emotional peak of the day had suddenly turned to the frustrating valley of the present. In the midst of it, I looked toward the sky and had a little conversation with God. It went something like this: "God, you sure do know how to keep a fellow humble. I guess I should say thanks."

The moral of this story is very simple. To have a wife who loves you and to have a place to be a servant for those who need help is the highest form of honor.

Treat interruptions kindly.

They just may contain

once-in-a-lifetime

opportunities.

Forty-Seven

Prognosis in Perspective

Yesterday was Christmas Day, 2002. I received a surprise gift — it was a phone call from my old friend Reed Hill. His voice needed no clarification, I immediately recognized the same unique lilt that I remembered from the first time I ever met him. At that time, he operated a "Five and Ten Cent store," as they were called in those days, just a few doors up the street from my little office. The thing that makes this story interesting is the fact that it begins in 1951 (as he reminded me). I was a very young doctor, practicing solo from a very modest office. It consisted of a few rooms in the back of Anderson's Drug Store. Dr. Carl Anderson had added them on for me and provided them rent-free at first. My shingle was a small piece of tin tacked onto the door facing. My name had been painted on a rather inauspicious scrap of metal by Wade Drummond, the local sign painter.

On our first meeting Reed recounted his life story. He had recently moved to our town, Woodruff, S.C. from the beautiful little mountain town of Black Mountain, N.C. He had a beautiful wife, Geneva, and two children, a boy and a girl. He had just been through a thorough work-up at a very prestigious research institution, and as he put it to me, he had been sent home to die. His son Mac was a sophomore at Gardner-Webb College, and was told he might have to drop out of college so that he could take over the business, as Reed wasn't predicted to be able to work much longer. After listening to him, and for days after that, I was haunted by his hopeless tale.

Yesterday, Reed reminded me of what I had said to him on that day back in 1955. According to him, my only comment that he remembers was, "I'm just not ready for you to die yet." His reminder awakened in me the recollection of that day, long ago tucked in the backside of my memory.

Reed Hill is now ninety-three years old, and enjoys a quality of life that we could never have dreamed on that day so long ago. He would have been about forty-five years old at the time. I must have been about twenty-five. The prognosis (outlook) of yore was bleak indeed. We chuckled a little yesterday as we realized the comment, "I'm just not ready ..." Fortunately for him, doctors are not always accurate in their predictions. Maybe we should speak less, think more!

To get along with the story, as time went on, the diagnosis became clear. An article in the medical journal had depicted a patient with his exact symptoms. An experimental drug had been found. Reed had myasthenia gravis. The pieces all came together. Reed was willing to try the new remedy. It worked. Now, forty-eight years later, he still takes six pills a day of that medication. He no longer wears "crutches" to keep his eyes open, and no longer strangles in his own secretions.

Reed and I have clocked a lot of miles since that fateful meeting in the back end of the drug store. We have both grown old now, but both felt all the younger for having gone back in time to recall the beginning of this story. Two young men, one willing to try "one more thing," the other trusting in a brash young doctor, naïve enough to try that "one more thing." Without that trusting relationship, the prognosis for his life would have played out differently. Without his faithfulness, willingness and commitment to take six pills a day, I would not have received a phone call yesterday, and you would not be reading this true story either.

Life is made up of a kaleidoscopic montage of little things, not always apparently significant at the time. Sometimes they take place in rather meager surroundings such as the back end of a drug store. Yesterday, it was Christmas 2002, and Reed's call was a reminder that on the first Christmas something far more significant happened in the back of a stable — in a manger.

Thanks, my friend, for making that call, and for allowing me to share your story. The morals of the story are: to never give up, to never be afraid to try "one more thing," and to hold onto hope, no matter what.

Reed, you are living proof.

Forty-Eight

In Whatever Way I Can

This letter was written just minutes after learning that friends of over thirty years had lost their daughter to violent suicide. She was only thirty-one years old and was a beautiful young woman. The parents had not yet been allowed to see her. The forensic work took precedence over such personal needs. Many questions, tears, second-guessing were evidence of all things human. I had written this letter before I had a chance to talk with them. When we did get a chance to talk, this letter stared at me from the computer screen. Something inside of me said, "Ask them if they would like for me to read it." They said, "Sure." After reading it, there was a moment of silence, after which they asked if I would read it at her memorial service, which I did. You will just have to read it as a raw, unedited, and spontaneous example of friends trying to embrace each other in a desperate time of great need. They gave me permission to share it with you.

Dear Paulette and Bob,

David just shared with us the news about Robyn's passing. Obviously, we are stunned. Talking is not easy at times like this. The e-mail seems easier. You know that we love you very much. That being said, I feel like I would like to get in the boat with you and grab one of the oars. Of course, many well-meaning people (friends) will offer condolences, but they will fall on barren ground, for they are not wearing your moccasins. We go through stages of second-guessing, what if ... The problem with that is that it is not helpful. Also, it is not required of us. This "requirement" is self-inflicted. It tends to fight Robyn's self-inflicted action with one of your own. Two wrongs never make a right. This is terribly unfair. The culprit might well be that in the human coil we simply did not understand all of the facts of the case, since we were not dealt a full deck of cards at the time, so to speak. Hindsight begins to present itself in all of its glory, even bigger than life itself, but it is out of sync with the time warp of reality.

Here is where I have to lay down my angry and resentful gauntlet of Ego, and turn loose. At least share my burdens with a caring and loving friend, and with God. God knows that, as hard as we try to fix our problems, some we cannot, so He has to take over. They are, I feel, that Robyn is with Him and that she is happier now, because together they are already working out the details. Some of your previous problems have been replaced with the vacuum created by her absence now.

The human hurt is still felt, and that is how it should be. Perhaps the only solution to all of her struggles was not one that we, or Robyn, could ever come up with in the framework of humanity. Divine choreography, in the heavenly framework, is the only answer. God is forgiving, more so than humans.

I will talk to you soon.

Love to both.

— Lewis

Sometimes out there ... in practice ...

you only have your head, your hands and your heart.

The outcome of the case depends on

how well you coordinate these three.

— *BLB, 12-4-71*

Forty-Nine

She's Never Been

This true story starts one morning in the first examining room on the east hall in our clinic. I had arranged to see Marcie first thing, since she and her husband Bill had driven straight through from Florida because she had a sudden episode of severe abdominal pain. They were determined to get back home so that she could deal with friends, not strangers. Upon entering the room with its very irreverent bold orange paint, I found Marcie lying very uncomfortably on the examining table. The paper covering crinkled audibly as she could not be still. I quickly went about to engage myself with taking the history. She had been on vacation in Florida, and out of the blue she was struck with pain that bent her double. I received a phone call that they were "on their way." As I then examined her abdomen, I found it to be soft, all sounds were normal, no history of intestinal abnormalities. My basic laboratory studies were all normal. I thought with Marcie aloud as I went. With every utterance of normalcy, I heard a soft voice from the corner. It was the voice of her husband of many years, saying, "She's never been like this." For the next few minutes, with repeated efforts to find some physical sign of the problem, Bill kept saying, "She's never been like this."

In my frustration and my own need to know just what it was that "had never been like this" before, I agreed to order an ultrasound study of the abdomen.

The report came back. Much to my surprise, the radiologist stated, "I believe there are some enlarged periaortic lymph nodes." This was the first such ultrasonic finding for me. A follow-up with more intricate studies revealed the diagnosis to be lymphoma in the biopsied nodes.

Marcie then underwent chemotherapy. She responded miraculously to such treatment. Now, many years later, she writes that her present doctor gave her "high marks" in all areas. This all because her loving husband kept whispering from the corner — "She's never been like this." In Marcie's last letter she says, "I do remember Bill saying those words. He was so mystified that I should ever be sick!"

Bill has since died after a long illness — Alzheimer's. Marcie was a faithful wife until the end. In the letter she added this addendum ... "When at the end he could barely put two words together, the last thing he said to me was, 'You're gorgeous.' What a sweet man!"

Yes, Marcie, he was that. His love for you saved your life.

Fifty

The Night the Brakes Went Out

The year was 1959, and I was nine years into my rural practice in upper South Carolina. I was proud of my sporty red Mercury Turnpike Cruiser with the gold streak down the side. It had successfully carried my wife and me on our honeymoon the year before, and was easily spotted throughout the county at all hours as I drove it on house calls.

This particular night after finishing house calls around ten o'clock, I drove into the driveway and parked uneventfully in the garage. After eating a belated, warmed-over supper and reading the paper, I went up to lie down for a while. In those days, I never expected to sleep through the night. Sure enough, a little past midnight, Molly Green called to say that she was in labor and on her way to the hospital. Since I only lived a short distance from the hospital, I lay back down and waited for the nurse to give me the details upon her arrival.

The phone rang and it was the night nurse at the small hospital. She was a fixture there. She was short, and a little more than a tad overweight. Her assessment was that Molly was about five centimeters dilated. It was not her first baby. Before I could get my clothes on, she called back, "You better come quick, she's bulging." Due to the urgency in her voice, I rushed out, cranked up the trusty Turnpike Cruiser and off we went, down the holler and up the hill to the hospital. Granted, I was in a hurry and slammed on the brakes. What brakes! Up over the curb and into the brick-veneered side of the building we went. The wall bowed and plaster inside fell. I had very specifically hit the nurses' lounge. Would you believe that my corpulent nurse was seated on the commode for a quick rest stop before the baby came, when the crash came? She was indignant at the intrusion of her privacy.

I rushed in, leaving the car partially in the nurses' lounge, and arrived in time to deliver the baby boy. I recently saw him on a trip back to that town. He is forty-ish and graying around the temples, very distinguished looking. Needless to say, he has his own embellished story about *the night the brakes went out.*

Fifty-One

Artist in Overalls

On one of our visits to our mountain cabin, which rests on the crest of the eastern continental divide, I noticed that the young trees in front of the deck had once again grown too tall. At least, they were partially obscuring the "million dollar" view of the Blue Ridge Mountains, including the picturesque Craggy Mountain chain, Clingman's Peak and Mount Mitchell.

I put in a call to my friend Robert Hart, an authentic born and bred mountain man who has never seen a problem that he couldn't fix. If he can't, he always knows some buddy who can. He is the man I count on when I need a helping hand.

This particular morning he came up to our mountaintop, armed with a chain saw (of the ordinary variety) and also a saw up on a pole. I think it is called a "topper." He was clad in a spiffy pair of Lee overalls.

He and I stood on the deck so that he could see what I "wanted to see." After a time he took the steps down to the steep, thickly overgrown terrain in front of the cabin. He was out of sight, but I could hear the rustling that his overalls made as they confronted the vines and briars. Then the cranking noises of the chain saw started. First one tree fell, then another, and another ... on and on the drone of the saw told the story of the clearing. Each time revealing an ever more beautiful site. Now the near mountain, Chestnut Ridge, came into view. With each buzz of the saw, the views slowly evolved and became more spectacular. Never on canvas had I seen such a sight. As any good artist would do, Robert came again to stand on the deck to eye his masterpiece in the making. He seemed never quite satisfied; again and again, he would return to what was the laborious task of using every muscle to lift the "topper" high over his head, just to clip a pesky top limb. With each bit of fine tuning, the extra effort was just in the right place to complete his masterpiece.

Now as I stood on the deck, surveying the wondrous 180-degree scene, my thoughts turned to the weary little man in overalls who was climbing up the mountainside. He was struggling at the weight of his heavy equipment.

My emotions overwhelmed me, and my feeling was that Robert had done a beautiful thing; his saws were his brushes, his canvas was furnished by God, and standing before me was ... an artist in overalls.

MARRIAGE

Marriage is like a beautiful bud at first. Through the years the bud slowly opens more and more. The full radiance of each petal must be experienced at the proper time. It does not appear at once. Then when the bloom is full, the feelings of appreciation are full. Then and only then, even the brown and falling petals can be understood.

— BLB

WHAT LOVE IS NOT

Love is not *all* physical attraction
Love is not *all* mental adjustment
Love is not *all* social alikeness
Love is not *all* spiritual agreement
Love is not *all* intellectual calculation
Love is not *all* financial security
Love is not *all* beauty
Love is not *all* desire
Love is not *all* in the present tense
Love is not *all* closeness
Love is not *all* your own
Love is not *all* sexual excitement
Love is not *all* maturity
Love is not *all* comfort
Love is not *all* for one.

But if it is found, it IS the common denominator
For two people, and the result is dual happiness.

Written March 17, 1958, just twenty-nine days before I gave
my beloved the ring, and proposed. Now it has been almost
forty-four years.

Fifty-Two

May Day, 1974

This is a story that I have needed to write for a long, long time, but I have never been able to. The reason is that it is so intimately close to home. It involves my father and me, in a place that neither would have chosen. My wife and I had just finished building our dream house on a fresh water lake in Mount Pleasant, S.C. Spanish moss decorated the huge live oaks that surrounded the property. My parents had come down to inspect it and on the way had experienced a flat tire, which taxed my father since the weather was already getting hot in our part of the country. My mother couldn't help since she had suffered from congestive heart failure the Thanksgiving before (while I was at home for a rare visit, by the way). They arrived, a bit exhausted, but were excited to see the new house. We were proud of it, they could tell. That made them happy.

On the Wednesday night, May 1, 1974, my father suddenly became dyspneic (short of breath) and began to wheeze. Fortunately, one of my residents, John Mitchell, and a student, Bill Brearly, were there with me. My family was at church. My father was suffering from pulmonary edema. He suddenly ceased to breathe; the heart stopped. John and I immediately began CPR (Cardio-Pulmonary Resuscitation). Bill was calling 911. About this time my family came in from church to see what was taking place.

I remember some of the details, but not all. I was doing what I was taught, almost by rote, as if I was in automatic pilot; so was John. The craziest thoughts kept coming through my head. My mother was on the floor in one corner of the room, crying her heart out. I knew her history at Thanksgiving; I happened to have been there then, too. (My friend, Dr. Bud Workman, had come quickly to help me then). The thoughts kept coming. I couldn't seem to stop them. What if your mother went into failure? Who do you love the most? Would you leave your father and go to her? How do you plan a funeral? These were strange thoughts whilst doing the task at hand. I would never have guessed that such diversions would plague my efforts. Did I break a rib? I would gladly toss this beautiful house in the lake if only this had not happened. God, why me? Then, God, why NOT me?

This was the first day that the EMS had operated east of the Cooper River. (Mount Pleasant is separated from the city of Charleston by the two-mile long Cooper River Bridge.) They got lost trying to answer Bill's call, finally coming down the wrong lane of a split boulevard to our house when they found their way.

By this time we had established a pulse and respirations. The paramedics rushed in, placed a rather crude respirator on my father's chest, and loaded him in the emergency vehicle. John jumped in to ride in the vehicle. He reported later what happened on the way across the long bridge. The respirator broke! The crew stopped at the first hospital that they came to, St. Francis. Bill drove me right behind. When the doors swung open at St. Francis, "they" quickly took my father in, but stopped me at the desk. "Are you a member of the family? "Yes." "Do you have insurance? Social Security number? What denomination is he?" On and on it went. "Who's your doctor?" In my distraught condition, I fear I had little patience with this scenario.

After my father's transfer to the Intensive Care Ward, Dr. Allen Johnson, another friend, came to our rescue. He took very compassionate charge of the details, which were out of my control. The long process of healing was on its way, but tedious at every turn. *My Dad,* I revert back to what I called this man when I was a little boy since I had been reduced to feeling that way in the midst of all this. I wanted to cry, but somehow knew everyone was looking at how I behaved. After all, I was a professor at the Medical School. I was, first of all, human. Why couldn't I cry?

This happened in 1974. I finally get around to writing it in 2002. It still hurts to think about it. I am so grateful to those who helped him, and me, then. The emotions were so scrambled at the time. I realize that I am not the only one who has had to weather such pain. We are not alone and we need to understand that regardless of whose moccasins we are wearing, it is extremely personal for all of us. I can say to others now, "I understand."

For years afterwards, my dad would ask me on just about every visit, "What happened, son?" After a silent, thoughtful moment, I usually said something like this: "Well, Dad, you gave me life once, and I tried to give you life once. I think you might have had more fun doing it than I did." He always smiled, then we talked about other things. He lived until November 7, 1980.

It is better to die trying to live

than it is to live trying to die.

— *BLB, July 15, 1987*

Fifty-Three

The Dancing Girl

I had made the trip down from our home in Virginia to my birthplace in the upper part of South Carolina. The purpose of my visit was to see my aging mother. She was in her nineties and "lived" in a private room at the end of the hall in the small hospital there. I approached the hospital with memories of my last visit there. I remembered that the only thing I could think of to do was to trim her nails. My mother had not recognized me and it hurt. One never wants to lose contact with the mother you knew as you grew up, the mother who shed tears when you left home, and the mother who shed tears of joy when you married, and when she welcomed grandchildren. So today my heart was heavy as I entered the lobby and started down the hall.

About halfway down the hall one of the doors was open. As I passed it, I heard someone call, "Hey, Doc, come here." I turned and made my way to the bedside of Willie Barton. His first question was, "How's your mother? We used to go to school together. She sure was pretty. We all called her the 'Dancing Girl' — Boy, could she dance!" He caught me totally off guard. He knew my mother before I did, and he had memories of when she loved to dance.

By this time, we had created quite a commotion along the hall, and others knew that I was there. Woody Abbott, the local druggist who was himself a patient, came out and added his recollection of my mother being "so nice" to him at the bank. She had been a bank teller in her productive years (to help send me to college).

I finally reached her room at the end of the hall. I quietly went in to find her resting. I bent over, kissed her cheek, and as I did, she opened her eyes. In that moment there was a clear sparkle in her eyes and a knowing expression crossed her face. I said, "Mom, I love you so much." She moved her lips and whispered "Do I." I believe those two words meant "I do love you, too."

As I left the hospital after my visit and walked toward the parking lot, I realized I had seen "the dancing girl."

Fifty-Four

The Only One ...

Virginia was a woman in her sixties, fraught with serious breathing problems. I saw her regularly in acute respiratory distress, asthma attacks so severe that she often ended up in the intensive care unit. Over the years, I found out a lot about her situation in life. She lived alone in a trailer. It was not in a very desirable place. Her children were not very kind to her. They only visited when they wanted her to take care of their children. Whenever there was a row in the family, which seemed fairly often, Virginia was sure to have an attack. No mention was ever made of her husband.

Each time she would get better, she seemed very grateful. She was unable to work at any gainful occupation. On one occasion, I was totally surprised when Virginia brought in a handmade quilt and gave it to me as a gift. It was made of hundreds of scraps of various colors of cloth. I hardly knew what to say. It is now about eight years later and we still have the quilt.

One morning as I was making rounds in the hospital, there had been a little boy admitted during the night with an asthma attack. His name was not one that I immediately identified. As I entered the room, a voice from down between the beds caught my ear. It was Virginia. She said, "This is my grandson, please make him better. He just had to inherit the wrong things from me, I guess."

Then she pulled out a picture from her over-stuffed hand bag. It was a worn and tattered Christmas card picture of my family, grandchildren and all. I had sent it to her with a note of thanks for making the quilt for us. It had become worn from her handling. She had been showing it around the ward. I was touched. I was touched even more when she looked up and said, "It's the only one I got."

As it did that day, my heart still sinks every time I think about it now. "The only one I got," indeed. I keep thinking and wondering how many folks that we meet are like Virginia and how we can tell.

Fifty-Five

The Therapeusis of a Rocker

I recently was up at our cabin on top of the mountain near Black Mountain, North Carolina. During that visit I spent some time in one of two cane-bottomed rockers that have been there for over thirty years. As I rocked back and forth, back and forth, I was aware that I had a much different feeling when it came to my appreciation of this fine piece of furniture. With each rock I was mesmerized into the subject of rockers.

I thought and day-dreamed, that rockers allow you to gallop, to trot, to jump the hurdles. You generally always stay in motion while sitting in a rocker. You can straighten your back, sit up straight, and go marching along while standing still, as it were.

The rocker makes you want to be active, while the cushy recliners of the world encourage you to do nothing. The rocker gives one a tether to the past, unlocking vibrant younger memories, creating a rhythm of regular cadence to life as it is now. That regular cadence, back and forth, back and forth, seems to welcome this time in life where the rocker is our friend. A friend that we somehow have time for now.

Fifty-Six

Fireworks

It is the Fourth of July, Independence Day. My wife and I are sitting on the front row waiting for the fireworks to begin. This year we are in the little mountain town of Black Mountain, North Carolina. We have had a little redwood cabin on top of Allison's Ridge, just south of town, for thirty-three years now. Our children have grown up knowing about this place. We have grown old clinging on to it. So many memories of together times were born here.

The spot we have picked to watch the "Big Show" is filling up with excited young folks, as well as a lot of us older folks. We remember Thomas Jefferson, but the kids may not. Asking when the fireworks will start, the answer is "when it gets dark!" Of course, I should have known that. And when dark came, sure enough, one at a time each rocket spread out overhead. They came one at a time so we could savor each as it made its own statement in the sky. A little lady with a unique red cap sat in the car beside us. Her license plate read "KERLEE B." I was told that she was eighty-eight years old and from one of the families who settled Black Mountain. She had her little dog with her — and she was the driver of this vehicle, out after dark. This was a big event. She leaned her head out the open window to get full view of each glowing burst of color. In a small town, if you listen, you will hear a lot about the place. In this case, I learned that her name was really Lucille, and that she was one of the "feisty" ones, still full of life and of "herself." She was not bashful, I could tell, because she had no thought that I was a stranger and carried on a banter that was as authentic to the area as were the mountains themselves.

After about forty-five minutes of enjoying the one-rocket-at-a-time experience, the grand finale came with a surprisingly spectacular array of light, sounds and smoke that told how close we really were to the site that "the town" had picked to set them off. With a flourish, it was done. The smoke lingered. This year's fireworks was different than any we had ever experienced before. It included not only the sights of light, but also the sounds like bombs bursting in air, and the smells of fire and smoke all around much like war itself. It was an altogether more intimate touch with the meaning of what we were there to celebrate — our independence and those who fought to gain it.

At the very end, when all of the smoke had cleared, in the cobalt of a crystal clear night sky there came as an encore a very awesome sight. In stark contrast to all of the man-made hoopla, there was an elegant, breathtaking full moon, all by itself. Lucille and I both agreed; that was the best part of it all because it was God's message that He still had a better way to do things "than we humans do."

We started to leave, but offered to let her go first, which she refused. Patiently she said that she wouldn't get in that crowd. They are always in a hurry. I am afraid she is right again.

Fifty-Seven

The Anvil Stands

In thinking about the *principles* at work in the practice of Family Medicine, I am reminded that they constitute something indestructible, something for the ages, something not bounded by time, something that shapes us, and something that never changes.

The image that comes to mind to encompass all of this is the *anvil*. The anvil is the everlasting tool that survives many a pounding. It helps to shape molten iron despite intense heat and constant battering from many hammers. The anvil/ the principles have withstood trials and hurts.

If we look to the future of Family Medicine, I am encouraged by the vision I have of this metaphor, the anvil. I see the image of the anvil in the center — with thousands of broken hammers piled high around it. The broken hammers represent all of those skeptics, doubters, reformers and changers who would rob us of our souls.

End of story: They will not succeed! The anvil stands.

Fifty-Eight

While Eating Supper

One summer night as I was sitting at the table having supper after a rather tiresome day at the office and hospital, the phone rang. Somehow the phone usually knew when I sat down to supper. My wife answered, trying to give me time to take a few bites. She handed me the phone, saying this is long distance.

As I swallowed a partially chewed morsel, I said hello. A crackling sound struck my ear, and through it came a familiar voice. It was that of a patient whose mother I was also treating. I asked, "Polly, where are you?" She replied, "I am on my yacht in the North Sea just outside of Copenhagen." This put a new meaning to "long distance." She was on a boat in the North Sea, and I was eating supper in my kitchen in Charlottesville, Va.

She was concerned about her mother. She wanted to know what I thought since I had seen her the day before. We talked, via satellite, for more than a few minutes. After being satisfied, she cheerfully bade me good-bye. I finished my supper.

My thoughts turned to what had just transpired. There was a satellite, a ship, the North Sea, a voice, wireless communication, many trappings of our modern world. But in it all, I wondered what it would all be worth, if the voice on this end had not been the one she wanted to hear. All of the technology in the world would have been worthless. Somehow, it is hard to even contemplate what this world would be without the personal human element that connects us all together.

Fifty-Nine

"Water Marked"

This profession has been ever so surely watermarked by Family Medicine. What is a watermark? It is an almost invisible marking on the finest of stationery. It needs only to be held up to the light to become clearly evident. It bears the hidden symbol of quality. It unashamedly and proudly announces who made it without boasting. All of this is true, but nevertheless, whether we see it or discern it or not, it is there. It is forever etched in the product on which all of history is written. You are a part of that history – you may be written over by high technological pieces, but never can be erased. The watermark of medicine – called by any name you wish, but the personal, quiet, unsung and sometimes invisible doctor — is always there.

WATCHING THE SUNRISE

A time of awakening, early morn,
listening to the winds;
West to east they blow
trees bending as if in
the posture of prayer.
Clouds blanket the mountains;
there is power in the winds.

Water standing, glistening
on the redwood deck
of our cabin in the sky;
The winds, the sun cast
a shimmering sparkle on droplets
left from a pre-dawn rain.

Sun casting a rosy hue,
contrasted now with clearing blue;
Sound of air currents gusting by
ranges of mountains
become bold in the distance.

Now the sun reigns over it all,
casting an icing on top
of the covering clouds,
much like a cake, a birthday cake,
celebrating the birth
of another new day,
a Gift to the world, and
all of us in it.

The valley below, still covered
by a soft cloud blanket,
does not yet know
that high above
the dawn has already come
to the mountain tops.

Such makes one want to shout,
to tell that another new day
has just been born.
Thank you, God
Your presence is palpable,
Speaking of majesty in it all.

Pointed peaks seem to mark
the very spot where
Heaven and earth touch,
and all of this and more
is a gift, it's free.

Being here now, a priceless time,
a priceless gift.
A sunrise, so quiet.
leaving so little doubt
that God is here, too

— *Lewis Barnett*
December 28, 2000

Sixty

Benjamin

This is the story of Benjamin, our youngest grandson. Yesterday was his third birthday. You see he is special — our miracle boy, we say to ourselves in our most private thoughts. I must explain, I know, because you can't understand unless and until I tell you more. So, as the Good Book unfolded, it said ... In the beginning ...

Our daughter Kristen was with child, her fourth, about six months along. The doctor ordered an ultrasound evaluation. The report was shocking. The doctor broke the news as gently as he could. "The heart has two defects, the intestines are obstructed, the placenta is too small, the fluid is too scant. The baby cannot live to term. If it does, it will be stillborn. Do you want to terminate?"

With this abrupt report, Kristen drove herself home and shared the report with her husband Jim and then called us. Strange as it may seem to some, there was no question that they would continue the pregnancy and try to handle it the best that they could. Their strong faith led them to know that God was in charge of their lives and also of this little one, too.

As the weeks passed, there was an ultrasound every ten days (for surveillance only). The first unusual happening came when the doctor said, "I can't believe it, but the heart looks normal!" Weeks passed, more ultrasounds, "The intestines have opened up!" Then, "The placenta is still a little scrambled and small, but it is holding on." At thirty-eight weeks gestation the report was, "The baby has stopped growing. We must induce labor." This was begun, but no sooner had it begun, Kristen began to bleed profusely. The placenta had separated prematurely. A crash Caesarian section was done, but not before her hemoglobin was down to seven grams (about half normal). The little fellow came through all of that, weighing in just over four pounds, crying for air and life. He wanted to live — he was a survivor!

I look at him now and know that surely he is here for some special purpose. Benjamin — that's my first name, too — and am I proud to have him bear that name. As I write this, I remember the day last summer when the family was at the beach together. Ben went to sleep in my arms with his "swimmies" on after exhausting himself in the pool. As I looked down on his peaceful face, I had no trouble understanding that I had the privilege of — holding in my hands — a precious miracle — named Ben.

Sixty-One

Writing in the Margins

Within a few days I will be seventy-six. I find myself living in an impatient world. Maybe more so now than ever, I feel the throbbing impatience all around me. Suffice it to say, I am now old. The racing cars driven by our young folks, by those late for work, passing me by, always honking, going around left and right, always going through yellow lights — often red ones — talking on cell phones, primping their hair, eating as they go, frighten me. Go-cups are the order of the day — subwoofers are packed in their trunks shaking the earth and vibrating your car as well as theirs, even two lanes away. I am sure they can't hear sirens or honks from others. Forbid that you stare or look at them. They are on edge deep down underneath it all. There seems to be no peace, no calm, no patience, even for those of us who need it. So I am writing in the margins, I guess. Just making pencilled notes in commentary to express how jangled it feels to me "out there." How did we get in such a stew and when will it ever end? For some it ends abruptly, tragically — and for them I weep.

Sixty-Two

One January Night

It was a very cold January night, about midnight, when the phone rang. On the other end was Evon Green, who worked in one of the local textile plants. His distressed voice beckoned me to come, "My wife is bad sick, please come." I crawled out of my warm bed and dressed warmly for the journey.

When I arrived at their modest home, it was dimly lit and cold. His wife was under many layers of quilts, and when you moved them they released an odor that bespoke fever and sweat. The slightest stirring of the covers caused her to shiver. The sheets were slick and in need of a good washing. There were very few choices of a place to sit.

A quick examination revealed that she had pneumonia. She was miserable. By the way, her name was Georgia and she was redheaded and freckled, but none of that mattered now. She became like every other human being in need of care.

The rest of the story takes place about twenty-five years later. I had left that small town to teach in a medical school. I revisited my little town and went by a Mom and Pop grocery store where I used to get "the best meat" when I lived there. As I was about to leave, the proprietor said to me, "Do you remember Evon Green?" I said, "Of course. I never knew another man by that name!"

The owner of the store continued. "He was in here the other day and asked me if I had seen you lately. I said no, but that you always stopped by here when you came to town. He related the story about one cold January night when you came to see his wife when she was badsick (somehow over the years bad and sick had become one word). He told of how I had put on my heavy coat to leave and turned to look at him as I started out the door and asked him, 'Evon, do you have enough money to buy the medicine?' He said I told him no. I gave you the last seven dollars I had. With a big tear streaming down his face, he said, 'He gave it back to me.' "

I relate this because I had forgotten about it until I was reminded. Sometimes in the middle of a cold January night, you do things and then forget. The subtlety of just doing what is right, at the right time, for the right reason is what life is all about.

Sixty-Three

Candle in the Wind

Just recently the entire world listened as Elton John sang one of his songs at the funeral of Princess Di. As I listened, this metaphoric sentiment seemed to resonate into an even bigger sphere than just a eulogy to one person. To me, it spoke to the way most of us exist — fragile, in the need of shields to protect us from the winds facing us whichever way we turn in this sometimes self-induced stressful society. Sometimes I think we manufacture our own problems — conjure up our own "winds" as it were. So many of us, seeking so many ways of coping. Sometimes we seem to face each day oblivious to the fact that we all need each other. It is amazing that the very shields to protect us from the threatening winds are all around us. They are our family. They are our friends. They are our beliefs. They do not hide the light of our candle; rather they buffer it against extinction. All of the nurturing that we need is within a touch — why can't we understand it?

The answer to that question is probably because we have come to worship too many secular gods — money, intellect, science, philosophy. Maybe we have tried too hard to create our own set of rules that define what's right and what's wrong. We say we are in the search of truth, but lose our way when we try to define it. Yes, we are very much like candles in the wind. The Greeks had the word "pneumos," which embodies both our words for wind and breath. So we can feel the winds that blow, but we can also feel life that comes from breathing. It then seems to leave it to us to figure what kind of God gave us the breath of life and also the shields to keep the light burning in our candle.

LIFE CYCLE: AUTUMN, NOW WINTER

It is Christmas Eve, the day
before Christ's birth.
Ice, sleet, snow abound.
A walk down by the creek;
Cold, very cold it is,
field coat and gloves,
appropriate gear for the trip.
Careful, calculated journey
on the stone staircase
created for just such days.
Safely now on the banks
of an active, lively, rushing stream.

Everything else is
frozen, still and rigid.
The fallen leaves of autumn
crunch beneath my feet.
The boots remind me
of warm feet, thanks to them.

Suspended animation, except
not so with the creek.
It bubbles and blows its vapors
over the rocks, the rough spots,
as it makes yet another statement:
bold, about life itself,
regardless of how rigid and cold.
The creek stayed not still enough
to freeze and become hardened
even if all else does.

Its struggle through the rough spots,
its foamy topping announcing
its victory on the other side.

The stream, which heralds life —
our lives, is vital and active,
moving on its way
to somewhere else,
perhaps to freshen and encourage
as another sits beside its banks.

— Lewis Barnett
Christmas Eve, 2000

Sixty-Four

Like Joseph's Coat

I had been warned by Professor Grumpen's wife that he had made his first appointment to see me, and that he had symptoms relating to every organ system. Furthermore, he just loved his old doctor in their previous hometown. She had built such a negative case for him that I almost dreaded to meet him. That day arrived all too soon.

Our first greeting was pleasant enough. I had braced myself and said a little prayer for patience before I went into the room. I had determined to listen, take one thing at a time, and to do the most thorough hands-on physical examination I had ever done (or at least as good as any). As he began to recite his multi-faceted symptom complex, I thought of the many colors in Joseph's coat. His history was just that color-ful. His biography became very interesting. My hands touched every part that he symptomized.

In the end, he got up off of the table, and as he arranged his clothes in the obsessive, meticulous fashion that you might expect, I sat down at my desk, assumed a very thoughtful posture, and waited — wondering just where to start. After an appropriate silent pause, I decided to say, "Professor, I don't know whether you feel better or not, but I sure feel better than when we started. You see, I was expecting to find something horrible and mysterious. Instead, I understand what you told me and can empathize with your frustration. But I think I left no stone unturned and am more able to relax now. You are basically very sound."

With this, he said, "Well, if you feel better, that makes me feel better. We can just process each problem as it comes along, can't we?"

The goodbye was with a handshake and two smiles — one his, the other mine.

Sixty-Five

Nostalgic Aroma

Some aspects of life we cannot see, we just experience them. This is such a story. It dates back a few years and is intimately personal. As I share it with you, my own life story becomes a little more transparent. I open it up. The warning is that if you allow yourself to think back in your own experience this story may touch you, too.

We received a late night phone call from our daughter Kristen telling us that our little grandson Will was in the Cobb County Hospital (GA) with a severe case of Respiratory Syncytial Virus and was struggling for breath. Her husband Jim was post-op from very recent knee surgery. She had not slept in days. With all of this, my wife and I grabbed a few essentials and set out from Charlottesville (VA) toward Atlanta. We drove all night and arrived just as the sun was thinking about coming up. After a quick stop for breakfast, we went directly to the hospital. There I went into the restroom and quickly shaved and splashed on my usual Old Spice Shaving lotion, as had been my habit since age 16.

We went up to Will's room and found both he and my daughter asleep. She was curled up in a chair next to his bed. He was in a tent with moisture and oxygen, making ominous sounds. I decided not to wake them — I knew that sleep and rest meant more than anything. So we tiptoed out and went down to the lobby to wait for the sun to finish its job. Not long after that, Kristen came rushing down to the lobby. After loving embraces, I asked, "How did you know we were here?" With a smile, reminiscent of when she was a little girl, she said "I smelled the Old Spice — Daddy's here."

Sometimes life is a series of connected memories, tucked away somewhere until we need them.

Among other things, this speaks to the utter humanity of the physician. We are real people with feelings, too.

Sixty-Six

Feelings of the Heart

Donald Vann, full-blooded Cherokee artist, said, "In our world, there is an unspoken quality, a feeling that touches and flows through everything — all of us, as well as all things of the earth. If one listens to the forces, he will find himself painting instinctively with the feelings of his heart, about his ancestral beliefs, and the way his people live today." So it is with us this day. It behooves us to try our hardest to hold on to the best of the past while trying also to relate to our present uncomfortable, modern-day predicament.

I find myself thinking about the soul of my profession — the wholesome goodness that brought warmth, while in the act of being a servant, sharing life with others from the stance of simple, purposeful living. The soul of our profession is that part which no one can claim ownership of — not the doctor nor the patient. It touches the shared existence between doctor and patient. It is that part of our profession that has been woven into a textured common denominator with our patients so that we are constantly aware of our reason for existence. God forbid that we lose this awareness — it is the antidote for burnout and dissatisfaction.

Sixty-Seven

Roller Coasters

All persons have many teachers along the way. They do not all have sophisticated degrees, or even know just when they turn into teachers. This true story is about a young man who for his sake I will give the name Max Johnston. The name is the only part of this story that is fictitious. We became acquainted after he had been brought into the emergency room. The history revealed that he worked in the sewage treatment plant in the Sanitation Department for the county. He had fallen into one of the enormous treating vats for the local sewage. How low can one get? The biography gradually revealed that he was the son of one of the distinguished professors at the university. He had left home and currently lived alone, except for a couple of cats. The scratches on his arms attested to their close relationship. He was combining drugs and alcohol even at work. This, I am sure, caused his loss of equilibrium and the fall into the vat.

Over the course of the next few months, many very intimate conversations took place in the inner sanctum of the confidentiality of a doctor's office. I picked up one oar, while I told of my expectation that he would pick up the other. I told him that there was just so much I could do, but I would do that. I expected him to meet me halfway. The conversation went like this. I said, "You do not have to continue coming to see me, but I care about you and I am never going to shut the door. You can always come back, and you are welcome." Then I did what some might never want to do. I wrote on a card my home phone number and told him my line would be open to him if he ever thought he needed to talk.

To shorten the story, I will say that he now makes rare visits just to tell me that "we made it through" and "thank you for not turning me away." I still get annual Christmas cards, always saying thank you.

He taught me something. He said that most all drug addicts or alcoholics have a risk-taking nature. They live life on the edge. They know that what they do is probably life-threatening. They do not respond to sermons. They are lonely. They may make friends of their risks. He now has replaced his risk-taking behaviors with seeking his thrills and his highs by traveling around the country to find the most daring roller coasters. He helped me to see anew and realize that I needed to understand this element of the problem — they need to feel a little thrill in life, to be a little higher than the average person does. His way of solving his need makes some sense once you accept his theory. Yes, we keep on learning, from the most unexpected sources.

THE MELODY OF LIFE

A tale about the melody of life
If all sounds were the same
and there were no choices of different notes,
there would be no music — only monotonous noise,
For you see, it takes variations to create music.

We are all different for a reason
because the world needs musicians.
It is full of those who hunger, who need
the peace of soothing melodies,
our melodies,
maybe no one else's.

Different notes,
variations on the theme,
one's distinct personality.
You
have a place,
your place,
in God's great scheme.

Predictability may lead to boredom.
Rituals and sameness likely
leave no surprises and make for dullness.
Dullness brings on constant hibernation
of the soul.
It can't come out to play
nor can it be kind and helpful
or separate from the self.
Others
cannot feel it.

Monotonous humming is an annoyance
much like ringing in the ears.
It produces no melody — no song.
Monotones, monotones — so little buoyance,
so little contribution, help!

Sometimes
one's difference
is one's contribution.
No effort to be negatively different,
no adversarial spirit,
just a resounding uniquity
belongs to no one else.
Here for a purpose, a reason —
music, a melody, a song
to be enjoyed by all.
Speaks to what makes life fresh, beautiful,
not just for self,
but for everyone.

— *Lewis Barnett*

Sixty-Eight

The Eyebrows Say Yes

Terry was a patient in the Hospice unit. He was forty-four years old and was suffering from Amyotrophic Lateral Sclerosis. Some call it Lou Gehrig's Disease; others remember Morrie Schwartz. He was totally paralyzed except for a few signals that went to controlling the small muscles around his eyes. I was making rounds with a very conscientious resident. As we entered the room I noticed a very attentive sister. The condition of his skin was most impressive — so smooth it glistened as the rays of the sun came through the window. Terry's only way to communicate was through charts on the wall and the help of his sister. She would point to the charts while he responded by raising his eyebrows when he meant yes and moved his eyes from side to side for no. The rest of his body was motionless. His feet were out from under the sheet.

As I stood by his bed, I felt an overwhelming sense of wishing and wanting to do something for him. The case was hopeless as far as affecting the disease, but here lay Terry Sanders, a nice guy, who had been dealt a nasty hand in life. I began to talk, and as I talked, my hands touched his feet. I grasped them gently, but positively. That touch reminded me of the characteristics of this disease. I said, "Terry, I know it is tough where you are. This disease is not fair. One thing about it is that it takes away your motor functions so that you can't move, but it does not affect your sensation. You can feel my hands touching." With that his eyebrows raised up (yes), and his eyes brightened. Something happened. What was left of his expression changed. Another human being had connected and understood. All we had to offer Terry that day was understanding and connection — not leaving him alone with his disease.

We left the room that day, knowing that he would not live much longer. The young doctor and I walked slowly down the hall on our way to the next patient. He was aware that something had happened back there. He had never really thought about the way this disease so selectively affected the motor nerves and that it does not rob one of the capacity to feel, so that touching is not only appropriate, but is the only thing we had to offer that day.

TRUSTEE OF DREAMS

Every day you have a chance to do something
that makes you feel wonderful to be alive.
To be a scientist, yes;
To be an artist, yes;
To be a priest, yes;
To be a confidant, trusted friend, yes;
To be the trustee of dreams, yes;
To live a life bigger than one's self.
That includes others, yes;
To be the owner of a happy pleasant kind of fatigue,
Having striven and become weary
is to be heir to a very special part of space
which connects us to all others
in a way that blends us
into the fiber of mankind
and leaves us standing,
clutching to our breast ...
Peace.

Sixty-Nine

Wren at My Window

A little over a week ago, I was surprised with a visit from an old friend. He happened to be in town for a meeting. He drove up to the door and parked his rental car and came in without knocking, as he was accustomed to doing over the twenty-plus years that our friendship covers.

The weather was beautiful outside — sunshine, crisp fall air, but giving no distractions to the warmth and rekindling of the seldom chance for the two of us to forget ourselves and live in what we used to call the "us."

You will most likely know the feeling I describe when I say that it seemed as though we took up where we had left off when we were together the last time. We were "at home" again with each other — one more time. It seems to me, now that I'm getting into the golden years, along with every day becoming more precious, that each visit also becomes more precious. Does that make sense to you?

Our relationship started in 1976, I believe. It began in Charleston, South Carolina. I was on the faculty at the Medical School there; he was an aspiring young doctor who was there as a resident in training. Many memories flooded my mind as we sat in my study — among them being the time he carried me home in his vintage Mustang when I had a rip-snorting attack of what later was obviously an attack of cholelithiasis (big word for gallstones). He was put into the precarious position of scrubbing in on my "big" operation which revealed 500 gallstones that had caused jaundice and,

I'm told, required five and a half hours on the operating table to flush them all out of the ducts. Having gone to the operating room with the thought that I might have pancreatic cancer, this was the fellow who yelled through the fog of the groggy post operation state to say, "It was gallstones, NO cancer." I had been on the other side of this equation all of my life. THIS was the fellow who was there as I was waking up. That mattered a lot.

But other more pleasant memories crept in as the sun sparkled on his now graying hair which reminded me again of my own advancing years. The happiest vision was of another such sunshiny day, Easter it was, in 1977, April the tenth to be exact. That was the day that I was given the gift of delivering their baby. He reminds me that my first words were, "She has such bright eyes." Now, twenty-five years later, they are still very, very bright.

So life can best be defined as a continuing series of blessings, joining with friends along the way and gaining nourishment from each other. The secret, it seems to me, depends on how much enjoyment one gets from seeing other people happy. This requires an entirely unselfish spirit — no one knows exactly how much of a boomerang that brings about, but I think it's a blue chip part of life.

As we sat, I could see out the window to a nearby Japanese holly (the tall variety), and suddenly a tiny Carolina wren lit on the most visible branch. What a healthy sign, I thought. You see, this friendship I have been sharing with you began in South Carolina twenty years ago. The Carolina wren is the state bird. We are in Virginia. This visit was not planned — it was unexpected. Was it a coincidence that the wren at my window picked this day to visit? Anyway, the little bird added warmth and helped rekindle the embers from the past. Yes, now I have yet another memory to cherish — the wren at my window, a very small, composite symbol of a ton of memories.

Seventy

You Are a Keeper, My Friend

This is a very personal story, mainly because Fred McCormick, a long-standing, rather complicated patient, became my friend. This so often happens in a practice that covers many years. Fred and I had gone through many ordeals, subtle subliminal manifestations of what I had come to call "McCormick Syndromes."

On this occasion, my friend became very ill. His major problem was coronary artery disease for which he had had a bypass done twelve years ago. Now the dragon was back. He was subjected to another battery of diagnostic tests and subsequently another (re-do) bypass. Just an hour or two back in the intensive care unit he went into shock. He had a pericardial tamponade (bleeding into the sac around the heart). This necessitated opening him up again right in the unit. The story becomes tedious and long. I was visiting him frequently during all of these scary episodes. He recognized a familiar voice. He clung to the trust that he had developed over the years. His anemia was corrected by multiple transfusions. He next developed a pesky resistant pneumonia. In his exhaustion he called his wife in, as well as his only daughter's husband, to tell them that he was ready to go and that he could fight no longer.

My visit this particular morning was somber. Fred said, "Lewis, it's over. I can't fight any more. I have given it my best. I give up. I'm ready." As I stood beside him, there was a silence, except for all the machinery around us. Two men, holding onto each other with the entire grip he and I could muster. As I spoke, the first words were, "You say you have given up." His weak answer, "Yes." My question, "Do you want me to give up, too?" After a long pause came the answer that my old Engineer Professor would naturally give, "Well, I will have to think about that." With that, my comment to my friend was, "I think you are a keeper."

Out in the waiting room I found his wife and daughter, weeping softly, appropriately. I recounted our last few minutes in the intensive care unit. When I told her that I had told Fred that I thought he was a keeper, she sobbed more openly, but she, too, grasped my hand.

Having given him time, "time to think about it", I returned to his bedside. "Have you thought about it?" His sunken eyes barely opened. He said, "I don't want you to give up." The ensuing hours and days were a struggle, but struggle he did.

I just talked to him by phone. He now is gaining strength and weight. He has a lilt in his voice, and he talks about a purpose for everything. He has been an inspiration to many — doctors, nurses, medical students, friends, church folks and anyone who has heard even a part of the story.

Yes, Fred, my friend, you indeed were "a keeper."

IT IS OKAY TO CRY

Tears are not always sad or happy,
good or bad, strong or weak – they are
merely the moisture of life itself like
the dew of refreshment and one of the
elements that awakens us to the
realization that we are human. Tears
prevent the soil of our existence from
becoming an arid desert where
nothing grows and where
understanding another's need is not
possible. Tears bathe and cleanse the
soul. It is okay to cry.

Seventy-One

On the Doorstep

I came home very tired one night not long ago, only to be met by my wife who said, "Let me tell you something. I had lunch with my friend Joan, and if you never did anything else in your whole life, this should make you feel that it's been worth living. Joan said that her daughter, Paula, told her the other day that if it had not been for you, she would be dead." (Paula has a husband and two children — she was at the brink of suicide). I suddenly felt a lump in my throat — I whispered, "Thank God." Yes, life in this profession is worth living. Amid all of the roller coaster moments, there are highs as well as lows.

Just a few days before Christmas that year (December 21,1996, to be exact), I found a package at my door. It had been left there unannounced and lay at my feet quietly. I reached down and picked it up. As I did, I noticed that there was an envelope underneath it. I opened it and began to read:

Dear Dr. Barnett,

It occurred to me that I've never taken time to tell you what I have thought many, many times — and that is "thank you." Somehow a simple thank you seems terribly inadequate to say to someone who saved my life, and more importantly, my marriage and any hope for happiness and normalcy that my children have ...

By now my eyes were blurred with tears ... She went on:

Your compassion, understanding, and wisdom have kept history from repeating itself and ruining another generation. I hope you know how grateful I am.

This story started with what her mother had related to my wife. It ends with the rest of the story. It leaves me with tears in my eyes once again, gratitude in my heart, and knowing now that the greatest gifts are sometimes found on our doorstep.

Seventy-Two

Ode to the Stethoscope

Please respect and appreciate your stethoscope and realize what it stands for and what it allows you to do. Treat it gently and handle it with reverence. The most difficult part of retirement and the hardest thing I have yet had to do is to lay the stethoscope down after a long, long romance with it that covered fifty-five years. So, do not take it, and the profession it symbolizes, for granted. There are those who are trying to tear down such gracious symbols. You are now the standard bearers, the guardians of the light and warmth embodied in this old friend, the stethoscope. Even though it often caused me to hear sounds that I did not want to hear, it also caused me to touch and to bend over.

The stethoscope has so long been a part of my life. You see, I have been a doctor since I was twenty-two years old, and now I am within days of being seventy-six. The intrigue of diagnosis, the soothing palliation of diseases, assisting in the improvement of the quality of life, the gift of being present as a player in the healing process gave meaning to daily encounters with one's fellows. To give it up, to retire, to quit as it were, would announce the ultimate arrival of life without the stethoscope, a strange kind of grief. It would be the giving up of what had been the source of shared joys and sorrows, the possible purpose for living.

So, my young friends, carry your stethoscope close to your heart, for although many techniques will try to replace it, none will.

Seventy-Three

Bill's Symphony

I have a friend (patient) of long standing named Bill. He has also been my "general contractor." We live in an old house built shortly after I was born, so, like myself, it needs a little TLC from time to time. If Bill can't fix it, he says we need a "specialist." That usually costs more money, as it does in my profession.

Bill is what we call in the medical profession a general practitioner. He also has become my friend. We talk from time to time. He has about two dozen dogs. We had only one, but she got old and down in the hind quarters and could not get up. We worried about what to do, but Bill came to the rescue. He related a story about what happens when a friend's favorite dog goes beyond the limit of good life. He says a friend comes by and takes the dog "home" with him. So that's what happened, and now Ginny is at peace. Now I know a new definition of what a friend is.

Friendships are daily, and needs change back and forth — never one-sided. The other day Bill came by and said, "I can't hear. I can't hear the alarm clock, but that isn't the big problem. (You see, he is what I call a Big fox hunter. That's really why he has all of the dogs.) Fox hunting assumes great priority on many fall and winter nights. As Bill interprets life in his world, he relates that he knows some "high-falootin' " folks like to listen to Bach and Beethoven, but with a gleam in his eye he says, "But listening to my dogs chasing a fox is my music. That's my symphony." So here again, Bill helped me with yet another definition of music appreciation. It makes it very important for us to see what we can do about his hearing. After all, there are all kinds of symphonies playing out there, and the quality of life depends on whether we can hear them.

Seventy-Four

Yeah, I'd Jump Again

This is the story of Lewis (a namesake of mine, by the way), a fellow I delivered when I was in country practice some forty-plus years ago. He did not breathe when he was born, but after much resuscitation, he came around. His first breath was mine, since mouth to mouth resuscitation was the method employed. His cry became music; his mother's cry was for joy; the moisture in the physician's eyes was forgivable. I told his mother at that time that he was very special. I told her that he was obviously here for some special purpose. Little did I know what was to follow. When he was sixteen, he jumped into Lake Greenwood, not knowing that the level of water was dangerously low. He sustained a broken neck. He has since been quadriplegic. Many members of his family enter into this story. His sister had married a man who was not very well accepted by the family. She and her husband had not been home for a long time. His older brother had majored in Spanish (and is now a professor at a major university up east), quite a ways from home.

One Sunday I went back to my hometown to visit and went to church. Across the auditorium I saw a wheelchair — Lewis was there. After the service was over, I made my way across the room amidst many warm embraces, but wondered whether to extend my hand to Lewis. I wasn't sure he could respond with his. As I got closer, Lewis made a very difficult effort to offer his hand to me. So I reached out to him. An emotional touch took place — I told him what I had said to his mother when he was born — that he was special — that he had a purpose in life. He stopped me short and said, "I know, I know. One of my therapists asked me, 'If you had it all to do over again, knowing what you know now, would you jump again?' I told her, 'Yes, I would jump again.' "

I listened closely to pick up his quiet voice as he continued. "Because it brought my sister home, my brother is part of the family again, and it got my daddy to the front of the church when he rolled me up to thank all of the kind people that showed us their love. Yeah, I'd jump again!"